THE
AGING
WORKFORCE

THE
AGING
WORKFORCE

Realities, Myths, and Implications for Organizations

Jerry W. Hedge
Walter C. Borman
Steven E. Lammlein

American Psychological Association
Washington, DC

Published by
American Psychological Association
750 First Street, NE
Washington, DC 20002
www.apa.org

To order
APA Order Department
P.O. Box 92984
Washington, DC 20090-2984
Tel: (800) 374-2721; Direct: (202) 336-5510
Fax: (202) 336-5502; TDD/TTY: (202) 336-6123
Online: www.apa.org/books/
E-mail: order@apa.org

In the U.K., Europe, Africa, and the Middle East, copies may be ordered from
American Psychological Association
3 Henrietta Street
Covent Garden, London
WC2E 8LU England

Typeset in Palatino by Stephen D. McDougal, Mechanicsville, MD

Printer: Bookmart Press, North Bergen, NJ
Cover Designer: Knoll Gilbert, Cincinnati, OH
Technical/Production Editor: Harriet Kaplan

The opinions and statements published are the responsibility of the authors, and such opinions and statements do not necessarily represent the policies of the American Psychological Association.

Library of Congress Cataloging-in-Publication Data

Hedge, Jerry W.
    The aging workforce : realities, myths, and implications for organizations / Jerry W. Hedge, Walter C. Borman, and Steven E. Lammlein.
        p. cm.
    Includes bibliographical references and index.
    ISBN 1-59147-319-5
    1. Age and employment—United States. 2. Middle aged persons—Employment—United States. 3. Older people—Employment—United States. I. Borman, Walter C. II. Lammlein, Steven E. III. Title.

    HD6280.H43 2006
    658.3'0084'6—dc22   2005007023

Contents

THE
AGING
WORKFORCE

Introduction

The Aging Workforce examines the changing demographics of the workforce and their impact on the world of work. The number of older individuals in the United States is fast increasing, as is their proportion in the population and the workforce. Most organizations are ill prepared to meet the challenges associated with older workers, and little research has been done to address the development and implementation of effective human resource (HR) management practices for an aging workforce.

The "graying of America" requires that we give more attention to both the problems and potential of an older workforce. Consequently, work psychologists should invest considerable effort in examining more closely the propensity for work in the aging workforce and in understanding more clearly the capabilities, motivations, interests, and expectations of this ever-increasing proportion of the labor force.

We believe that the timing is right for a book that pulls together research findings relevant to individual older worker performance and offers suggestions for how best to manage the older worker. With a mix of the academic and the practical, the book provides a "state-of-the-science" perspective on what we know about issues related to the older worker, thus providing a foundation for confronting the challenges facing the workforce of the future.

Given the centrality of work in the lives of most individuals, we expect that the aging workforce will have an important impact on the world of work. Therefore, we attempt in this volume to provide background, data, and useful insights into a fascinating and ever-evolving phenomenon. In the chapters that follow, we address issues of age stereotyping; age discrimination; research on aging and physical capabilities, cognitive abilities, job performance, attitudes, and personality; job trends and the aging worker; and the relationship between various HR practices and the older worker.

As the nation's 78 million baby boomers (those individuals born between 1946 and 1964) age, the number of older Americans will skyrocket. Relatively few baby boomers are confident they will have enough money to retire; a majority of 48- to 56-year-old individuals are behind on planning and saving for retirement, and many have no retirement savings at all. Those who have not saved for retirement are not likely to get immediate help from Social Security, because the eligibility age for full benefits is increasing in steps and will reach 67 for those born in 1960 or later. It is not surprising that many older workers say they expect to retire far later than age 65, perhaps in part because medical science has increased life expectancy in the past 50 years, and consequently, retirees will need to fund more years of retirement than ever before (Wellner, 2002).

After the baby boom, the birth rate dropped sharply. This "baby bust" resulted in fewer entry-level workers after the mid-1990s and is likely to lead to similar shortages in mid-level and executive talent in the decades ahead. Consequently, older workers will form a significant and largely untapped labor pool whose appeal to employers is likely to increase, as happened in some industries that faced shortages of entry-age workers in the 1980s. In chapter 1, we examine some of these demographic trends and what they mean for the world of work.

In chapter 2, we review the role that ageism plays in the workplace. Older workers face widely held societal stereotypes that manifest themselves in ageist attitudes and age discrimination. We examine these factors within the context of the Age Discrimination in Employment Act (ADEA; 2004) and underscore the importance of the proposition that management must adhere to the spirit of the law—that each person should be judged on individual merits and should be provided with equal opportunity to make the best contribution to the workplace and realize his or her aspirations.

Chapter 3 deals with the effects of aging on performance—physiological, cognitive, and job performance. The chapter highlights the remarkable capacity of older workers to adapt to age-related changes and maintain performance levels by adjusting their approach to the job. Chapter 4 addresses the notion that being successful in work and nonwork situations is a function not only of the individual's knowledge, skills, and abilities but also of certain noncognitive attributes. This chapter is concerned with (a) relationships between age and job satisfaction, job involvement, and organizational commitment; (b) the role of personality in older people and, indeed, across the entire adult life span; and (c) various coping strategies older workers might use to ensure personal and occupational well-being.

Chapter 5 takes a closer look at the changing world of work. Changing retirement patterns, changing occupational trends fueled by ever-evolving technological innovations, and changing motivations and capabilities of workers as they age mean the HR landscape of tomorrow will be vastly different and more challenging than it is today. To attract and retain sufficient numbers of employees, organizations will have to include older individuals in their workforce and must understand how older workers' needs and motivations differ from those of their younger counterparts.

All of these changes point to a need to develop strategies that better allow for successful integration of older workers into the workforce, and this is the focus of chapter 6. To optimize utilization of the older worker, organizational HR specialists need to gain a better understanding of issues surrounding older workers, including skill and knowledge obsolescence; the need for development of new, cutting-edge knowledge and skill resulting from technological innovations; and the importance of creating new opportunities for employment and motivating and rewarding different age groups in the workforce.

In chapters 7 and 8, we take a practical look at ways organizations can deal with an aging workforce. Chapter 7 discusses areas of concern for organizations that wish to better utilize older workers: targeted recruitment strategies, the processes of selecting and placing older workers in jobs, job redesign for older workers, flexible work alternatives, and flexible compensation and benefits. This is followed, in chapter 8, by an emphasis on the roles of training, performance management, career management, and retirement planning for older workers.

Regardless of the changes organizations make in the structure and functioning of the workplace of the future, it appears likely that older workers will play a crucial role. Organizations need to make it worthwhile for employees to continue to be productive and to gain satisfaction from their work activities as they age, which will lead to positive outcomes for both older employees and their organizations.

We have written *The Aging Workforce* for a diverse audience. Psychologists and business professionals will find useful information about such relevant issues as age-related stereotypes and literature-based findings about performance and motivation differences between "younger" and "older" workers. Supervisors and HR managers will be exposed to the latest thinking on how best to retain, use, and motivate older workers. Researchers will find a set of practical issues and unanswered questions to be explored across a wide range of content areas. Although our intent is to provide a state-of-the-science update on what the research has to offer about issues related to work and the aging worker, the book is not an academic treatise on the topic but rather a more basic work that we hope will be readily accessible to a large audience.

There are many reasons why people choose to write a book. The three quotes that follow provide some of our rationale.

> The list of major global hazards in the next century has grown long and familiar. It includes the proliferation of nuclear, biological, and chemical weapons, other types of high-tech terrorism, deadly superviruses, extreme climate change, the financial, economic, and political aftershocks of globalization . . . . Yet there is a less-understood challenge—the graying of the developed world's population—that may actually do more to reshape our collective future than any of the above. (P. G. Peterson, 1999, p. 42)

> Old people get older and usually less productive, and they ought to retire so that business can be better more economically served. We should treat the elderly with respect which does not require treating them as if they were not old. (Safire, 1977, p. 29)

> My friends are getting older, so I guess I must be too. (Brown, 1992)

Certainly, the changing face of the workforce mirrors that of the population, and promises to have a major impact on workforce effectiveness and efficiency. In addition, today there still exist many misperceptions and misunderstandings about what contributions can and should be expected from older workers. Finally, we are all aging workers and have a stake in how the aging workforce is changing the structure of work and retirement.

1

The Graying of the Workforce

The world's population is aging rapidly. In 2004, over 10% of the global population of 6.1 billion was at least 60 years old. Recent projections suggest that by 2050 this figure will climb to 20% and that those age 60 and over will outnumber children age 14 and younger. Similar trends can be seen in the U.S. population. In 1860, half of the population was under 20 years of age; half of the population was still under the age of 30 in 1950. In 2000, Americans age 65 years or older numbered 35.0 million, an increase of 3.7 million (or 12%) in just 10 years.

The U.S. population will continue to age in the future (see Figure 1.1). This trend, like many trends in the latter half of the 20th century, will be fueled by the large population cohort known as the *baby boom generation* (those born between 1946 and 1964). Even more rapid growth will occur between the years 2010 and 2030, when this cohort reaches age 65. By 2030, it is expected that there will be about 70 million older persons in the United States, more than twice their number in 2000. Thus, people age 65 years old and older will make up 20% of the population by 2030 (U.S. Department of Health and Human Services, Administration on Aging, 2001).

Preston and Martin (1994) have suggested that the rapidly aging population of the United States represents "one of the most important social phenomena of the next half century" (p. 3). They argued that eligibility for most major entitlement programs is tied

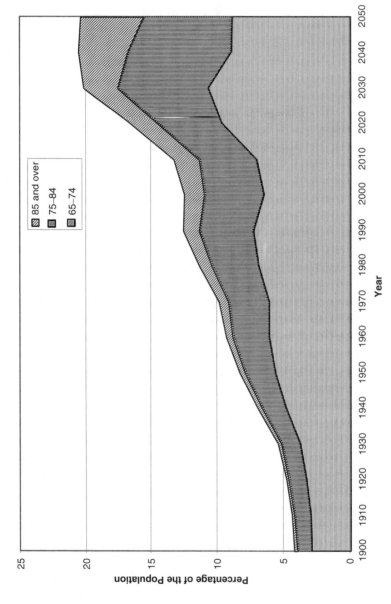

Figure 1.1. The aging population of the United States. Data extracted from U.S. Department of Health and Human Services, Administration on Aging (2003).

to age and thus is affected by changes in age population structures. Because these changes are mirrored within nearly all social
institutions—from families to organizations—how these institutions adjust to these changing demographics may have a significant effect on the quality of life in the 21st century.

Workforce Demographics

According to the Bureau of Labor Statistics (U.S. Department of
Labor, Bureau of Labor Statistics, 2001), nearly 13% of the
workforce was 55 years and older in 2000. Between 2000 and 2010,
that age group will increase to almost 17% of the workforce. Thus,
during the first decade of the 21st century, the number of workers age 55 and older will jump from 18.2 million to 26.6 million—
a 46% increase (see Figure 1.2).

Although the profile of the U.S. population and workforce continues to reflect a grayer tint, the participation rate for older workers consistently declined for much of the 20th century. At the beginning of the century, retirement was atypical, with two thirds
of American men over age 65 employed. However, by 1950, just
over 45% of men age 65 or older were in the labor force, and by
1990 that number had dropped to under 17% (see Figure 1.3).
Actually, this participation rate declined steadily until about 1985,
when it reached just under 16%; after that it leveled off and even
increased slightly, reaching 17.5% in 2000 (Fullerton & Toossi,
2001). A similar trend was evident among men between the ages
of 55 and 64, whose participation rate fell from just under 87% in
1950 to almost 68% in 1985.

As can also be seen in Figure 1.3, the labor force experiences of
women have been different from men's in many ways yet similar
in other ways. The participation rate of women ages 65 and older
has remained low, fluctuating within a relatively narrow range.
However, as noted by Fullerton and Toossi (2001), the participation rate of women between ages 55 and 64 has increased sharply
over the past several decades. As of 2000, almost 52% of women
between the ages of 55 and 64 were in the labor force, up from
27% in 1950 and 42% in 1985. Nonetheless, the rising labor force
participation rate of middle-aged women was not enough to
counter the decline among middle-aged men. Consequently, by

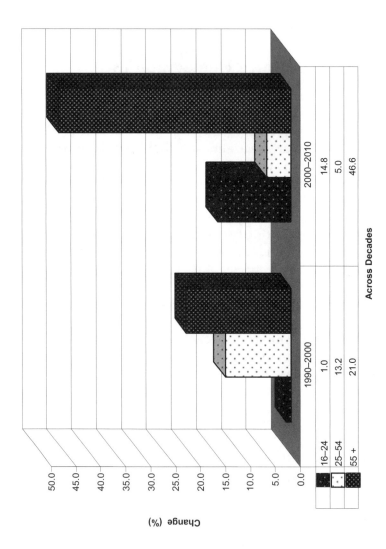

Figure 1.2. Change in workforce composition. Data compiled from *Economic and Employment Projections: 2000–2010* (U.S. Department of Labor, Bureau of Labor Statistics, 2001).

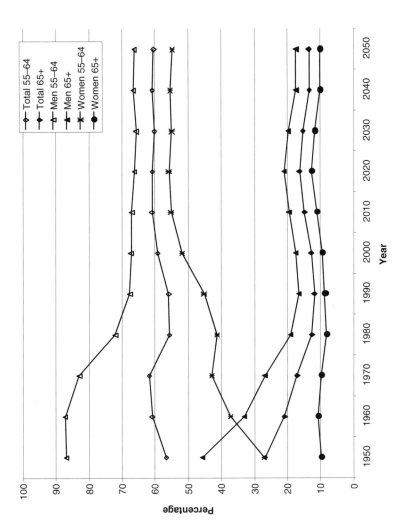

Figure 1.3. Actual and projected workforce participation trends. Bureau of Labor Statistics and Bureau of the Census data extracted from Toossi (2002, Table 3).

1985 just over 30% of the population age 55 and older was in the labor force, down from 43% in 1950. By 2000, the participation rate for individuals age 55 and older had risen to over 32%.

The trend toward increasingly earlier retirement, however, appears to have leveled off and begun slowly to reverse (see Figure 1.3). Looking to the future, the labor force participation rate among men age 55 and over is projected to rise by 4% between 2000 and 2010. Although it remains to be seen if this is a permanent change, growing numbers of men appear to be working somewhat later in life.

Obviously, demographers' ability to project future worker age profiles is dependent on many variables. Changes in any of these variables could cause the participation–retirement mix to change overall or to change differentially across certain occupations. Still, almost certainly impending shifts in the demographics of the workforce, along with important economic and workplace trends, have made the understanding of issues related to the older worker an increasingly critical area for both human resource practice and research.

In a recent report, Penner, Perun, and Steuerle (2002) noted that within the next decade the United States will begin to lose the services of millions of highly skilled and experienced workers as baby boomers begin to retire. This problem is exacerbated by the drop in fertility rates following the baby boom (often referred to as the *baby bust*), creating the potential for labor shortages. Therefore, it seems timely to examine the factors that might influence older workers to continue to contribute in the workplace and what might encourage them to retire. It is important to understand what is known about older workers' capabilities, interests, and motivations. It is also useful to become familiar with some of the age biases still prevalent at work and the legal protections offered older workers under the Age Discrimination in Employment Act (ADEA). These issues are discussed in detail in subsequent chapters as are many practical concerns related to hiring, training, and retaining a group of experienced workers who are becoming an increasingly larger segment of the workforce. Before moving on, however, we examine briefly some of the issues that older workers face as they ponder retirement.

Factors That Affect Labor Force Participation for Older Workers

The retirement decision is a complicated one, influenced by an individual's mental and physical health, attitudes toward work and leisure, social networks, living arrangements, financial resources, and expectations about the future (Quinn & Burkhauser, 1994). In addition, employer policies, national regulations, economic conditions, and job availability play a role. Withdrawal from the labor market is taken within the constraints of these institutional and personal factors. Discussion of some of these influences should provide some insight into the movement by aging workers into or out of the labor force.

Institutional Factors

Mandatory retirement. In the middle of the 19th century, American society was largely agricultural. Individuals worked on family farms until they were no longer able; then they stayed at home and were supported by their families. Even early in the 20th century, as the United States moved toward a more industrialized society, retirement plans among early factory workers were limited; people worked until they were no longer able or until they had sufficient savings to retire. Thus, a decision to retire tended to be based on health and wealth, not age (Rosen & Jerdee, 1985).

However, in 1935 the Social Security Act was passed as a means of opening jobs for millions of unemployed workers by providing income security for the older population once they left their jobs, and retirement at age 65 became the norm (Social Security Act of 1935, 2004). It is interesting to note that as described by Sheppard and Rix (1977), cultural factors rather than biomedical evidence were primarily responsible for the selection of 65 as the age at which full retirement benefits would become available from Social Security. Because of an abundant supply of young workers, organizations could easily "replenish" their workforce with younger and cheaper labor. In addition, employers often voiced concern about the ability of older workers to perform adequately in a faster paced, industrial setting.

Private employer-provided retirement benefit plans (when available) were often designed to complement Social Security. Of course, at that time average life expectancy was about 60 years, thus creating relatively short-term financial responsibilities for those entities that supported retirees. Subsequent changes in the late 1950s and early 1960s to retirement age benefits largely reinforced the 65 or younger retirement target. For example, Social Security introduced early retirement benefits at age 62 but kept 65 as the age for receiving full benefits; employer-sponsored benefit plans continued to introduce early retirement features, sometimes as early as 55 years of age (Wiatrowski, 2001).

Mandatory retirement rules once covered a relatively large proportion of the working population in America. In fact, prior to 1978, about half of all American workers were covered by mandatory retirement provisions that required them to leave their jobs no later than a specific age, usually 65. The 1978 amendment to the ADEA made age 70 the earliest possible mandatory retirement age for most American workers (ADEA, 2004). Consequently, employers had to amend their retirement benefit plans to eliminate involuntary retirement provisions prior to age 70. In 1986, the age limit was removed, eliminating mandatory retirement for the vast majority of American workers.

Not only did the increase and eventual elimination of mandatory retirement age improve the options open to older employees who wanted to remain on their jobs; according to Burtless and Quinn (2001), it also sent an important message to Americans about changing expectations for retirement age. Still, policy changes and broad perspectives on the appropriate retirement age do not change deeply ingrained stereotypes and beliefs overnight (H. L. Sterns & Kaplan, 2003).

The abolishment of a mandatory retirement age for most occupations (exceptions include jobs such as commercial airline pilots and air traffic controllers; legal issues related to such exceptions are discussed in more detail in chap. 2) allows older workers greater flexibility concerning decisions about retirement. As shown in Figure 1.3, beginning in the 1980s and 1990s, there was a shift in the labor force participation rates of older workers, with a greater percentage electing to remain employed. Because many workers used to target retirement at age 65, it would be logical to assume that mandatory retirement has been an important factor in the retirement decision. However, some research has suggested that may not be true. For example, Parnes (1988), using a large sample of American men who had retired by 1981, found that only 3% of individuals who retired at the mandatory retirement age preferred to continue working. Burkhauser and Quinn (1983) noted, however, that age 65 was also the age at which important Social Security and employer pension retirement incentives went into effect. They suggested that what looked like a mandatory retirement effect was probably due in large part to financial incentives associated with Social Security and private pension plans.

Downsizing through layoffs and early retirement programs. Until the 1980s, many people in their 40s, 50s, and 60s felt that they would have a choice about working beyond the normal retirement age. This expectation was based on a confidence in a strong economic climate. Consequently, many middle-aged and older workers were caught off guard by the large numbers of layoffs and early "buyouts" and the general trend toward downsizing that has become a favorite corporate strategy, even for companies experiencing current success in the marketplace.

Although older workers in the United States have some legal protection against age-based job loss through the ADEA (which is discussed in more detail in the next chapter), organizations using downsizing to cut costs have an incentive to remove older employees because they typically have higher salaries than younger workers. Chan and Stevens (2001) recently showed that in the United States, the probability of job loss increased most for workers ages 55 to 64. In addition, if the worker was 60 or older at the time of the job loss, the probability of returning to the workforce within 2 years following job loss decreased substantially. In fact, as Bovbjerg, Jeszeck, and Petersen (2001) noted, citing data from the 2000 Displaced Worker Survey conducted by the Bureau of Labor Statistics, 57% of older workers who lose their jobs retire, partially or fully, following a job loss. Thus, many of these older workers eventually "withdraw" from the workforce—they are no longer willing to actively seek employment and thus become "retired." Displacement and unemployment rates have grown faster in the 1990s for older workers than for other age groups (Farr & Ringseis, 2002).

Many companies in the past 20 years or so have used early retirement incentives to manage the size and composition of the workforce. Certainly, from a public relations perspective, companies tend to prefer decreasing workforce size through these early-out retirement programs rather than through layoffs. Although employers cannot legally force employees to accept early retirement, they may pressure them to do so. They can also make early retirement attractive by augmenting private pensions until workers become eligible for Social Security benefits. If such incentives carry a time limit by which a "go or stay" decision must be made, and workers cannot be sure that they will not be laid off at a later date anyway, the early-out package may prove too tempting to resist. Under such circumstances, the extent to which workers can be said to be retiring voluntarily is questionable (Rix, 2001).

Although the problem of personnel cutbacks is a complex one, employers often make the following assumptions about older workers when the early-out option is used:

1. Younger employees, with their careers ahead of them, stay longer than older employees.
2. Younger people are inherently more "able" to do the job than older employees.
3. Older employees are close to retirement anyway.
4. All employees want to retire as early as possible.

Such generalizations often lead to poor policies regarding early retirement.

Although early retirement incentives are often aimed at getting rid of higher paid older employees (as well as some low-performing individuals), they often result in some of the best performers opting out; the less productive employees try to hang on because of their limited ability to get other jobs. Consequently, using early-retirement options may eliminate the people with the greatest experience and organizational know-how, thus leading to reduced levels of productivity in both the short and long term (Shea, 1991).

Social Security. Several recent changes in Social Security retirement policy could increase the incentives for older Americans to remain longer in the labor force. First, the 1977 and 1983 amendments to the Social Security Act significantly scaled back pension levels for future retirees (Social Security Act of 1935, 2004). Workers who retired between 1950 and 1980 did so in an environment where Social Security benefits were rising faster than average earnings; this is no longer the case (Burtless, 1993).

Second, the age at which retirees can receive full Social Security benefits began increasing gradually in 2000. Under a provision of the 1983 Social Security amendments, the "normal retirement age" will rise from 65 to 67 by 2027. A third change to Social Security was the liberalization of the annual earnings test, which historically reduced benefits for those who continued to work while receiving benefits. In April 2000, the earnings test was scaled back, and now it only applies to individuals receiving early retirement benefits before reaching normal retirement age. Then, when normal retirement age is reached, full benefits are available, regardless of earnings.

Finally, Congress has also changed the Social Security pension formula to make work late in life more attractive. When this change is fully implemented, for workers attaining age 62 after 2004, there will be no financial penalty for delaying retirement beyond the normal retirement age. Still, as Burtless and Quinn (2001) have pointed out, numerous simulations of various Social Security reforms all suggest that their aggregate effects would be small—on the order of months, not years.

Private pension plans. Important changes have also been taking place in the private sector. Over the past 20 years, there has been a steady increase in the use of defined-contribution pension plans relative to defined-benefit plans. A *defined-benefit plan* generally pools contributions into a single fund, on behalf of all participants. An individual's retirement benefit is usually determined by salary and length of service, regardless of the investment performance of the plan. Thus, the plan sponsors (or for the public sector, the taxpayer of the sponsoring entity) bear the investment risk.

A *defined-contribution plan*, most frequently, places all contributions in individual accounts on behalf of each participant; the plan specifies contributions to be made, but the benefits are linked to investment performance. Defined-contribution plans are age neutral by design (i.e., not based on age or tenure), and therefore they have none of the age-specific retirement incentives that are common in traditional defined-benefit plans.

According to the U.S. Department of Labor (2004), private sector workers covered by a defined-contribution plan increased from 14.4 million in 1980 to 46.9 million in 1999 (a 225% increase), whereas those covered by a defined-benefit plan decreased from 30.1 million in 1980 to 22.6 million in 1999 (a 25% decrease). It is not surprising, then, that research has suggested that the pension effects, for those covered by defined-benefit plans, may have a much greater impact on retirement decisions than the Social Security incentives (Burtless & Quinn, 2001).

Duka and Nicholson (2002) suggested that the recent trend among employers away from the traditional pension plans and toward these 401(k)-type plans may keep many older people on the job longer. They noted that whereas 401(k) plans may be better suited to a mobile workforce than traditional pensions, they have shifted more of the risk to the worker, a fact that becomes all too clear during stock market declines. Unfortunately, defined-benefit plans are also not without risk, as demonstrated of late by a number of companies dropping their defined-benefit plans as part of bankruptcy proceedings (*The Pension Underfunding Crisis*, 2003) and news that companies with underfunded pension plans reported a shortfall of more than $275 billion in 2003 (up from $18.46 billion in 1999; Taub, 2004).

As millions of older people have seen their retirement savings shrink, more have concluded they will have to work longer to avoid outliving their savings. Korczyk (2002) noted that the current generation could be in greater danger of outliving their retirement savings than their parents were because they are more likely to be covered by these defined-contribution retirement plans. In fact, baby boomers will be among the first retirees to derive all or most of their private pension income (if any) from defined-contribution plans. That the current generation will have a longer life expectancy than previous generations will only exacerbate this situation.

These various public and private pension plan changes have no doubt altered the future of the retirement landscape. There is evidence that more changes will occur in the future, as new types of retirement plans are developed and issues related to Social Security are debated. Still, whereas private pensions are a growing source of income for retirees, a study by the AARP (2001) noted that only about one third of Americans age 65 and older receive income from a private pension, and this percentage has increased only marginally in the past 20 years. Also, according to Copeland (2004), only 42% of all workers participated in employment-based retirement plans in 2003. In addition, participation levels were lower for employees who were non-White, young, female, less educated, lower income, and less healthy; who had no health insurance through their employer; and who worked less than full time.

Health insurance. Although many industrialized countries provide universal health insurance to their citizens, such is not the case in the United States. Health insurance is instead included as part of an employer's compensation package for most American workers. However, Wiatrowski (2004) estimated that between 1992/1993 and 2003, the percentage of private sector workers participating in employer-provided medical plans steadily declined. Medical care covered 63% of workers in 1992/1993, but only 45% of workers in 2003. Some employers also offer continuing health insurance coverage after their workers retire, but such protection is shrinking, and many employers now require their retirees to pay more of the cost of the plans.

Health insurance is especially important for workers who are not yet eligible for Medicare but are past middle age, because these workers on average have greater medical expenses. Thus, workers with employer-supplied health insurance, who would lose it if they retired, have an increased incentive to remain on the job, at least until they become eligible for Medicare. Conversely, those with postretirement health benefits have less incentive to remain employed. As Quinn (1999b) noted, inferring the overall effect of health insurance incentives on retirement patterns is difficult, because wage rates, pension coverage, health insurance, and retiree health benefits tend to be highly correlated, and it is difficult to distinguish statistically between the separate effects of each component of compensation.

Still, given the rising importance of health insurance coverage to older Americans, we would expect it to have some impact on retirement patterns, although exactly what the impact will be is less clear-cut. On the one hand, increased health insurance costs for employers might create additional roadblocks for hiring and retaining older workers (although, as we discuss in chap. 2, recent court rulings may lessen this burden on employers, meaning that older workers may be more cost-effective). On the other hand, the need to maintain adequate health care coverage may encourage (or force) older workers to remain in the workforce longer.

The economy. One potentially important factor affecting retirement may be the state of the U.S. economy. In the second half of the 1980s and much of the 1990s, the economy was strong, with both steady economic expansion and employment growth. Certainly, an expanding economy makes it easier to find and keep jobs. Weak labor demand discourages jobless workers from persisting in their job search. Strong demand creates employment options for older workers who want to keep working. Still, Quinn (1999a) estimated the cyclical economic impact on older workers' participation rates and found that changes in the overall unemployment rate account for a relatively small proportion of the change in participation percentages.

Personal Considerations

In addition to institutional factors, many older Americans base their retirement decisions on personal considerations. Important among these are health considerations and perceptions about financial status in retirement. Not surprisingly, as noted by Farr and Ringseis (2002), planned retirement age decreases as health concerns and perceived financial status increase.

Health and the physical demands of work. Health is one variable that affects the ability of older individuals to work. In the 1940s and early 1950s, about 90% of new retirees cited poor health or a layoff as the reason they left the workforce. Less than 5% reported leaving because of a wish to retire or enjoy more leisure. Such retirement explanations dominated survey responses and the research literature through the early 1970s. By the early 1980s, however, the reported reasons for leaving began to shift, with nearly 50% of male retirees age 65 or older attributing their retirement to a desire to leave work; poor health accounted for only 20% and involuntary layoff about 15% of retirements (Burtless & Quinn, 2001). As P. B. Levine (1993) has pointed out, however, much of the data are based on self-reports, so it is possible that those who retire early may be more likely to report poor health because it is a more socially acceptable explanation.

As we discuss in greater detail later in this book, age-related changes in physiological functions do not necessarily translate into job-related shortcomings. One study found that 80% of the 65- to 68-year-old and 78% of the 69- to 74-year-old U.S. workers reported no limitations on the amount or kinds of activities they could perform at work (see H. L. Sterns & Miklos, 1995). Also, as noted by H. L. Sterns and Sterns (1995), although health problems are more frequently experienced by older adults, differences between younger and older adults are relatively small.

In addition, given the changing nature of work and the reduced levels of physical requirements, the physical demands of work are now easier to meet than they were in the past. This shift to a service economy and workplace changes have allowed some employees with health limitations to remain at work. In fact, Burtless and Quinn (2001) suggested that there is no convincing evidence that the health of 60- or 65-year-olds was declining between 1950 and 1985, a period in which older Americans' labor force participation rates were falling. Rather, declining mortality rates and downward trends in the physical disabilities of the aged suggest that the health of Americans is improving, at least in early old age (i.e., 65–74). Also, Newquist (1986) warned about the dangers of treating older adults as a homogeneous group; greater variability exists with the population over age 65 than in individuals under age 65. Consequently, reporting older workers as a single group tends to portray, for example, individuals in the 65–74 age group as less healthy than they actually are.

Financial resources. Burtless and Quinn (2001) have suggested that one of the simplest, but most straightforward explanations for earlier retirement is increasing wealth. Over the past 40 years, the real per capita GDP in the United States has more than doubled, and one way workers have used financial gains is to retire at a younger age. As noted by Wiatrowski (2001), retirement income is generally composed of Social Security, employer retirement benefits, and personal savings, with Social Security generally being the single biggest source of income.

As perceptions of expected financial income become less certain, the probability that many employees will want to work beyond traditional retirement age will likely increase. In addition, Czaja (2001) has noted that the declines in the real value of pension benefits and declines in retiree health care coverage create a need for many older people to return to work after retirement from their primary occupation. Even for those employees who can count on government pensions or on Social Security supplemented by private pensions or savings, there frequently is no assurance that retirement income will be an adequate shield against the impact of inflation (or disastrous investments). As a result, many older employees may be strongly interested in finding ways to sustain their real income beyond "normal" retirement age (Rosen & Jerdee, 1985).

Intrinsic benefits. Beyond issues of health and wealth, older adults may wish to stay longer in the workforce. Given that many older people are healthy and active, they may desire to continue working for what H. L. Sterns (1998) has called "intrinsic benefits of work." Older workers may be interested in developing new skills, using their time productively, and making useful contributions to organizations or society. In addition, the work one does contributes to one's identity and sense of self; work allows people to stay in touch with current developments, and older workers who have certain expertise may wish to take advantage of additional training in their own or related disciplines or to take on new challenges. People who enjoy work may want to continue to maintain the social interactions and relationships they have with coworkers and to feel that they are participating in meaningful activity.

Exit Patterns From Career Jobs and Postretirement Employment

Although we have briefly discussed factors that affect an older worker's decision to stay or leave the workforce, some attention should also be paid to the labor patterns of older workers after the conclusion of their career jobs. We have an inadequate understanding of why some workers choose to retire partially whereas others do not, why many workers choose to reenter the labor force following retirement, and what major barriers are preventing older persons from accepting part- or full-time work (Beehr & Adams, 2003).

Researchers have only recently begun to examine more closely the exit routes that older Americans take between full-time work and complete labor force withdrawal. Although many still make this transition in one step, others occupy one or more bridge jobs between the two. Despite the fact that most of the economic literature treats retirement status as dichotomous, Americans actually leave their career jobs through numerous pathways. A substantial number of Americans do something other than leave the labor force when they leave their career jobs. According to Shultz (2003), perhaps as many as one third to one half of older workers move to bridge jobs before full-time retirement.

Numerous surveys reveal interest in some form of postretirement employment, with a majority of workers saying they would like to continue working part time for some period of time. A comparison of the career and bridge jobs revealed that most of the transitions involved movement to different occupations and industries, often at lower pay and without benefits. In fact, for many retirees, the types of job offers available are at such odds with their job market aspirations that they may not even consider employment an option. There are offsetting advantages, such as flexibility of hours; different working conditions; and, for many, the ability to claim a career job pension when its asset value is at its peak.

Workers who retired might have preferred some alternative to full-time retirement, if an attractive one were available. It seems reasonable to assume that were the part-time options more attractive, the number of older employed workers using part-time work as a path to retirement would rise. Part-time work could serve as a means of extending the work life beyond what it might otherwise have been.

A concept that has gained increased attention of late is that of *phased retirement*, a process used to characterize the transition from full-time employment to full-time retirement. As noted by

Wiatrowski (2001), phased retirement may take a variety of forms, including (a) using retirees as consultants or as temporary, seasonal, or part-time workers; (b) reducing work hours gradually over time; (c) allowing employees to take "leaves of absence" while still employed, to "sample" retirement; and (d) allowing older workers to engage in job-sharing arrangements as a means of reducing work hours. Still, formal phased retirement programs are relatively rare in the United States (see AARP, 1999), and some question whether such programs amount to anything more than a way to turn veteran employees into a contingent workforce (Greller & Stroh, 2003). Nonetheless, the fact remains that a substantial portion of workers leave long-tenure or career jobs and enter what are referred to as "bridge jobs" or "transitional employment" for a period of time before full-time retirement.

Rix (2001) cited six reasons for the likelihood of increasing numbers of older adults in the workforce. First, she suggested that workers may not be financially prepared to retire at age 62 or 65, given the rising age of eligibility for full retirement and concerns surrounding the Social Security benefits improvements. Second, over the past 25 years or so, employer-provided pension coverage has leveled off at roughly half of wage and salary workers. Third, among workers covered by these pension programs, the percentage of defined-contribution plans has risen sharply, replacing defined-benefit plans that guaranteed a certain benefit amount throughout retirement. In addition, workers with defined-contribution plans face considerable market risk, as stock market activity in 2001 and 2002 so clearly demonstrated. Fourth, many workers lack much in the way of personal retirement savings. Fifth, continued increases in life expectancy may raise worries among workers about outliving their retirement savings. Finally, educational attainment in the older population is comparatively high, and because higher educational levels have been associated with a greater probability of postponing retirement, this factor may keep more workers in the labor force longer.

Conclusion

Healthy adults spend a major portion of their time and energy engaged in work activities. Thus, the world of work provides a structure to their lives by determining things such as the distribution of time, schedules, and places they frequent. In addition, personal interactions, prestige, and influence are often directly or indirectly tied to employment, as is the demonstration of aptitudes, skills, knowledge, competence, creativity, and attitudes (Forteza & Prieto, 1994). Our review of demographic trends in this chapter should underscore the need to rethink traditional workforce models that embraced the routine replacement of experienced, older employees with younger workers.

There are signs in the United States that the trend toward ever-earlier retirement that characterized the mid-to-late 20th century has not only come to a halt but may actually have reversed direction. In addition, changing organizational contexts—downsizing, redefinitions of the psychological contract, increased technology, and globalization—have altered employer and employee perceptions about the world of work. Consequently, it makes sense for work psychologists to invest time and energy in examining more closely the propensity for work in the aging workforce and in understanding more clearly the capabilities, motivations, interests, and expectations of this ever-increasing proportion of the labor force.

The changing work landscape also underscores the need to rethink and reshape employment and retirement practices to meet the needs of older workers and their employers in the 21st century. In this chapter we have tried to paint a relatively broad picture of these workforce and workplace trends. In the chapters that follow, we examine many of these issues in greater detail.

2

Age Stereotyping and Age Discrimination

A ge prejudice is one of the most socially accepted forms of prejudice in America today. According to Sheppard and Rix (1977), discrimination against older people is more ingrained in American minds than is sexism or racism. Whereas most responsible people and organizations now accept that race and gender cannot be used to judge occupational fitness, the movement to ignore age when making such judgments is only just beginning. Myths of aging are prevalent in our popular and professional literature, print and sound media, on Web pages, in conversations, and in jokes, and they subtly shape social, health, and work experiences (Nelson, 2002). Collectively, these aging myths create an image of aging and being old that is biased and damaging to the careers and well-being of older persons. Thornton (2002) suggested that the current myths stigmatizing aging and older people involve general perceptions that include being unhealthy, senile, lonely, grouchy, sexless, lacking vitality, and unable to learn or change.

Myths of aging are also found in a work organization's culture and are often reinforced by its policies and procedures. These myths influence the attitudes of others toward "older people." Unfortunately, older persons' perceptions and expectations of aging are also shaped by these myths, which potentially makes these myths a self-fulfilling prophecy. Rosen and Jerdee (1985) noted that in a business context, decisions based on race, sex, or age stereotypes run the risk of ignoring or misjudging individual differences in skills, abilities, and motivations. Such stereotyping may result in an underuse of human resources, to say nothing of the potential adverse impact on an individual's self-esteem. Moreover, stereotyping may lead to illegal differential treatment of particular employee groups. In summary, stereotypical thinking can lead to false impressions, poor judgments, and inappropriate actions.

Shea (1991) suggested that managers at all organizational levels may struggle when dealing with age issues because they lack clear information on the laws related to age discrimination and how these laws are applied in the workplace. These problems are often exacerbated by misunderstandings about the nature of the relationship between age and work performance. According to Faley, Kleiman, and Lengnick-Hall (1984), much of the sharp increase in the number of age discrimination complaints and lawsuits can be traced to managerial age-biased stereotypes as well as ignorance of the legal rights guaranteed older workers by federal and state laws.

The Age Discrimination in Employment Act (ADEA) aims to achieve age-neutral decisions by ensuring that hiring, promotion, training, education, and other personnel actions are not influenced by a person's age. The intent of the ADEA is to (a) promote employment of older persons based on their ability, (b) prohibit arbitrary age discrimination in employment, and (c) help employers and workers find ways to overcome problems arising from the impact of age on employment. As discussed in chapter 1, the "graying of America" represents a major challenge to the social, political, medical, and economic structure of society. In the current chapter, we discuss issues that may lead to age discrimination and provide an overview of the ADEA. Before proceeding, however, a brief discussion is warranted on what defines an "older worker."

Defining the Older Worker

The term *older worker* is commonly used, but there is much variability in how it is operationally defined. For example, the ADEA

(2004) designates age 40 as the legal demarcation of an older worker; the AARP uses 50 as the age of eligibility for membership; the Older Americans Act (1965), the Job Training Partnership Act (1982), and the Workforce Investment Act (2000) use "55 and older" as the definition of an older worker. Because 65 had been the traditional age for retirement and receipt of Social Security benefits, that age is frequently cited as the benchmark for becoming elderly. Indeed, it is not uncommon to see old age classified into *young old* (approximately 65–75), *middle old* (76–85), and *old old* (over 85). No wonder the term *old* is problematic.

Maurer, Wrenn, and Weiss (2003) noted that there are also no established age cutoffs in the age research literature. Definitions of what constitutes "old" vary considerably, from 35 and over, to 36–60, to 55–67, to 58–84; some use a median split to separate a group into younger and older adults. Adding to the confusion, many of these studies seem to lack any rationale for choosing a particular age to define a worker as "older." Simpson, Greller, and Stroh (2002) noted that often the age range is expanded simply to adjust for the decrease in the number of people in the "older" category. In a review of 105 studies that defined the term *older worker*, Ashbaugh and Fay (1987) found that the average chronological age as operationalized in research of an older worker was 53.4 years.

H. L. Sterns and Doverspike (1989) concluded that aging is a multidimensional process that is difficult to adequately depict in a single definition. They suggested that different levels of analysis are related to different aspects of aging and that one can choose to study individuals, organizations, or society. Consequently, some researchers have offered five approaches to defining older workers that provide discrete but related ways to conceptualize various aspects of aging. These perspectives on aging include (a) chronological–legal, (b) functional, (c) psychosocial, (d) organizational, and (e) life span. The life span approach borrows from a number of the previous approaches but suggests that substantial individual differences in aging are recognized as critical in examining adult career patterns.

H. L. Sterns and Gray (1999) suggested that although legal definitions and social norms provide guidelines for defining older workers, in truth, individuals use the age range that suits their own unique conceptualizations. The approximate age range included in one's conceptualization of younger, middle-aged, and older workers may vary with individual differences such as respondent age, age bias, and perceived retirement norms.

Age Stereotyping and Age Norms

Stereotypes are learned ways of perceiving and organizing the world that provide us with information that guides our interactions with others. They are affected by cultural, economic, and social factors; peer pressure; and even firsthand observations. *Age norms* are widely shared judgments of the standard or typical ages at which individuals hold a particular role or status (Lawrence, 1988). Such age stereotypes and age norms can have a significant influence on expectations of performance, the performance itself, and how that performance is evaluated.

Research on Age Perceptions, Stereotypes, and Norms

There is a small but growing literature on the influence of age perception, stereotyping, and age norms on age-related outcomes. These studies have examined issues like how age stereotypes affect managers' performance evaluations, how age perceptions affect selection decisions, and how age norms limit the work contributions of employees. For example, Cleveland, Festa, and Montgomery (1988) found that when a job applicant pool became more heavily made up of older applicants, the age stereotype of the target job began to increase as well. This would suggest that the job–age stereotype itself may be fluid and capable of being influenced by the demographics of the people in the applicant pool. Similarly, Cleveland and Hollman (1990) examined the age composition of incumbents and the age type of job tasks and found that as the proportion of older workers in a job increased, so too would the rating of a job as appropriate for older adults.

In another study, Gordon and Arvey (1986) examined the idea of occupational age norms. They asked study participants to estimate the average age of workers in 59 occupations and then compared these estimates with the actual ages of workers in these occupations. They found that individuals are relatively accurate at age typing different occupations. In addition, they found more variability in age perceptions for "older occupations" than for "younger occupations," suggesting that people find the latter easier to type than the former.

Cleveland and Shore (1992) studied the relationship between chronological age, perceived age, and job performance and found that age perceptions interacted with chronological age to account for more variance in job performance measures than chronological age alone. They suggested that the relationship between chronological age and work outcomes depends on the views people hold about age, and they proposed that supervisors' and coworkers' interactions with and evaluations of the worker are influenced more by perceptions of a worker's age than by the person's actual age.

Perry, Kulik, and Bourhis (1996) found that the nature of the job affects the extent to which biased raters penalized older applicants. Specifically, the older applicant was evaluated less favorably than the young applicant when the rater was generally biased and the applicant applied for a younger type job. However, when the older applicant applied for an older type job, he or she was evaluated more favorably than the younger applicant. These researchers suggested that the potential for age discrimination may increase as organizations begin to use video interviewing and video resumes in the selection process, at least in part because demographic information may become more salient and readily available earlier in the selection process.

A set of meta-analyses examined factors associated with age stereotyping and age discrimination. Finkelstein, Burke, and Raju (1995) conducted a meta-analysis of empirical studies examining age discrimination in real and simulated employment settings. They found that younger respondents judged younger workers as more qualified than older workers and believed that the younger workers had both a greater potential for development and were more physically qualified for demanding jobs. Younger raters rated older workers more favorably in terms of job stability, however (i.e., dependable, careful, steady). In contrast, older respondents in the study rated younger and older workers as equally qualified for employment. In a meta-analysis, Gordon,

Arvey, Hodges, Sowanda, and King (2000) found a small overall bias against older workers as well as a slight bias against older adults in terms of job qualifications and interpersonal skills. This bias against older workers increased significantly, however, for judgments of workers' potential for development. Conversely, older workers were viewed significantly more positively in terms of stability than were their younger counterparts.

Thoughts About Age Norms and Age Stereotyping

Lawrence's extensive research on age norms may help to provide some context for the pervasiveness of negative stereotypes about older persons despite evidence to the contrary. Recall that age norms are widely shared judgments of the standard or typical ages of individuals holding a particular role or status. These beliefs, shared by the organization's personnel, about what happens to people as they age in a work environment produce the age norms for that organization. Consequently, then, these age norms sanction and reinforce specific behaviors within a given social system, thus producing age-related patterns of behavior. These norms, in turn, often have a direct and adverse impact on managerial behavior toward the older employee. If, for example, the current perception in an organization is that workers automatically become less motivated as they age, a manager may feel that it is unnecessary to design incentive plans for older workers (McCann & Giles, 2002).

According to Lawrence (1987, 1988, 1996), society has expectations concerning the levels of success that should be reached by certain ages. For example, by the time that individuals reach their late 50s, society expects them to be in positions of seniority, and often authority, at work; anything less represents a failure. Similarly, people develop perceptions of what age milestones mark those who are on schedule, ahead of schedule, or behind schedule in their careers. As a result, age becomes associated with meanings of status and power that are based on the job an employee holds. Young people in "older" jobs (especially those who have advanced higher up in the hierarchy) acquire high status and power as a result of their age, whereas old people in "young" jobs tend to acquire low status and power labels.

By extending this line of reasoning to managerial evaluations, one might assume that when supervisors evaluate older employees against younger employees who may be viewed as "on a fast track," the supervisor's appraisal may be influenced by norms that dictate where in the organization each worker should be at his or her respective age. In terms of the theory, then, the supervisor might downgrade the older worker and upgrade the younger worker in performance evaluations (McCann & Giles, 2002).

Lawrence (1988) also suggested that the age distribution of old and young workers in a particular job helps to dictate the age norms associated with the job, producing an age-based timetable for that job. The distribution of chronological ages in a job has an actual "typical age" as well as age ranges representing the youngest and oldest employees. Because speed and extent of progression up a career ladder vary by job, some jobs have a wider distribution of typical ages than others. In addition, managers exert some control over job age distributions through selection and retention activities. In addition, Lawrence (1987) has shown that age norms differ across organizations; in fact, even in the same industry, organizations may develop widely different age norms.

Warr (1994) suggested that the important point about stereotypes is not that they are completely false but rather that people who use them often do not recognize that considerable variability exists within age categories and that an "average age" representative of a particular category may not be particularly representative. For example, the notion that people should retire at age 65 suggests that some milestone event occurs for all people when they reach that age. Sheppard and Rix (1977) emphasized the fallacy of stereotyping age groups and also challenged the use of averages (i.e., the idea that the "average" 60-year-old person can or cannot do this or that) in making decisions about a specific individual's capacity to perform in specific job tasks or the age at which an individual should retire. Thus, generalities about the capabilities of specific age groups—often the root of stereotypes—should be viewed skeptically. An individual's "functional" age is influenced by both inheritance and environment, a fact that suggests a fair amount of variability within age groups.

In truth, considerable variability exists both between younger and older employees and between people who are the same age. Forming impressions on the basis of chronological age alone while excluding other kinds of information often leads to inaccurate conclusions. Hummert (1999) suggested that age is a unique social category in that (unlike race or gender) individuals progress unavoidably from one category level (i.e., young) to another (i.e., middle age) to yet another (i.e., old) over time. Lawrence (1996) echoed this view of age as a social phenomenon and noted that whereas chronological age certainly carries considerable predetermined biological information, it is the meanings that people attach to age and the behavioral consequences of these meanings that are of interest.

Attitudes Toward Older Workers

Several studies have documented managers' attitudes and skills in managing an older workforce. For example, Rosen and Jerdee (1977) asked corporate managers to examine hypothetical organizational and personnel problems and to decide on proper courses of action. Although the respondents suggested that they valued both younger and older workers, their recommended solutions indicated a biased perspective. For example, whereas 31% of the participants felt that current business practices with respect to the treatment of older employees were inadequate, and 77% favored greater emphasis on affirmative action programs for older people, the personnel decisions they made as part of the study systematically discriminated against older employees. Rosen and Jerdee found that the respondents generally believed it was more difficult to change the behaviors of older workers and that items are best routed around them. The managers also did not attribute positive motives to older workers who desired retraining, saw older workers as less likely to be promoted than younger workers, and favored career development for younger workers over older workers.

Hansson, DeKoekkoek, Neece, and Patterson (1997) cited a study by the International Foundation for Employee Benefit Plans that found that although 86% of Fortune 2000 companies say they "value" older workers, only 23% have organizational policies that encourage the hiring of older workers (Capowski, 1994). Similarly, a study by Simon (1996) found that 55- to 64-year-olds received training opportunities much less often than did 35- to 44-year-olds. Rix (2001) noted that the AARP has periodically surveyed several hundred organizations to track the attitudes and perceptions of employers and their policies toward older workers. These surveys, conducted since 1985, have revealed that employers consistently tend to rate older workers highly when it comes to loyalty, dependability, experience, and customer relations; however, they rate older workers far less positively when it comes to flexibility, adaptability, technological competence, and ability to learn new technology.

Thus, although survey results show that employers give older workers high marks on certain characteristics, negative stereotypes of older workers persist among American employers. Perhaps in no other area is this perception more striking than in the area of training, where beliefs are strongly held that older people are unwilling to change, learn too slowly, do poorly in the classroom, are computer illiterate, and are not worth training because they will not be around long (Rosow & Zager, 1980; Simon, 1996).

To the extent that age stereotypes influence managerial decisions, there are potentially serious consequences for older employees, including lowered motivation, career stagnation, and job loss. Thus, when the new positions demand creativity, mental alertness, or the capacity to deal with rapidly changing situations, managers may make much less effort to give older persons feedback about needed changes in performance, provide limited organizational support for the career development and retraining of older employees, and limit the promotion opportunities for older people (Rosen & Jerdee, 1985).

Ageist clichés imply that specific behaviors are appropriate for each stage in life. As we have discussed, persons age at different rates physically, mentally, and so on. Consequently, people who belong to a specific age cohort become less alike as they grow older (Hale, 1990). Nevertheless, ever since the enactment of the Social Security Act, age 65 has become a marker of sorts for when older adults are officially (and unofficially) "sent out to pasture." Consequently, work may suddenly no longer be expected from those who have spent a lifetime devoted to their careers. Powerful age norms that dictate that age 65 (or younger) is the time for rest and relaxation have the potential to clash with the wishes and needs of older individuals (McCann & Giles, 2002).

Older Workers' Stereotypic Beliefs: Impact on Their Own Work Attitudes and Behavior

In a recent review of stereotypic beliefs about older workers, Maurer et al. (2003) suggested that through a self-fulfilling prophesy, stereotypes might also influence older workers' perceptions of what is appropriate or possible for individuals in their age group. They cited several studies to support this perspective. For example, Greller and Stroh (1995) suggested that stereotypes might influence workers' concepts of appropriate aging behavior, leading them to conform more closely to others' expectations. In addition, Hassell and Perrewe (1993) found that older workers who believed age discrimination existed in their own organization had lower levels of self-esteem and satisfaction with growth opportunities than those who did not. Similarly, D. M. Miller et al. (1993) found that older employees who perceived that there existed a belief by others in the organization that older workers' performance deteriorates with age and that younger workers received preferential treatment experienced low levels of job involvement and alienation from the job.

Maurer and colleagues also speculated that the extent to which older workers believe that their age group has more difficulty and is less interested in learning and development, is likely to affect their own beliefs about their ability to develop and the usefulness of learning and development activities. They also suggested that older workers employed in jobs requiring learning who tend to believe that aging workers are not capable of or interested in learning and development are more likely to retire sooner than older workers who do not have these beliefs.

Age Discrimination in Employment

Age discrimination can be accidental or intentional, subtle or blatant. According to the federal government, age-discrimination complaints filed with the Equal Employment Opportunity Commission (EEOC) rose more than 24% between 2000 and 2002. In addition, an average of nearly 16,500 age discrimination cases per year have been filed with the EEOC since 1995, a figure that amounts to roughly 20% of all cases filed with the agency (McCann & Giles, 2002). Table 2.1 provides an overview of cases filed with the EEOC between 1995 and 2003 and the monies realized as a result of these claims. These financial totals do not include money that has resulted from litigation actions but rather only those cases resolved prior to litigation. In addition, in 2003 alone, almost 24% of all cases filed with the EEOC were age related; these were the most frequent cases filed with the agency after race, sex, and re-taliation claims (EEOC, 2004).

With the vast improvements in medicine, nutrition, and lifestyle in recent years, it might seem like an odd time for age bias to be on the upswing. The problem is that workplace culture has, for the most part, stuck to old ways of thinking about older workers (Cohen, 2003). This way of thinking—and acting—has been ex-pressed in discriminatory practices such as (a) limiting or exclud-ing older workers from substantive job responsibilities and ac-tivities, (b) removing older employees from the workforce through negative performance evaluations or through encouraging their retirement; (c) implementing insensitive, poorly conceived poli-cies; (d) limiting older workers' access to job-related education, career development opportunities, or employee benefits; and (e) refusing to hire or promote older workers (Steinhauser, 1998).

The disconnect between workers who view themselves as pro-ductive and companies that view them as "washed up" has helped to promote this sharp increase in age-discrimination claims. In-deed, in many U.S. job markets (e.g., investment banking, infor-mation technology, publishing), youth is celebrated, and regard-less of how young older workers may feel, they only have to look around to realize that they probably are not viewed as part of the "new wave." In addition, the downsizing business trend that began in the late 1980s helped to focus attention on age discrimi-nation, given that it was especially consequential for workers over 50.

Some more basic social factors are at work, however. With the graying of America, there are simply many more people eligible for discrimination. There are more than 70 million baby boomers,

Table 2.1

Age Discrimination in Employment Act Cases Filed With the Equal Employment Opportunity Commission Between Fiscal Years 1995 and 2003

Fiscal year	No. of cases	Monetary benefit (millions)[a]
1995	17,416	$29.4
1996	15,719	$31.5
1997	15,785	$44.3
1998	15,191	$34.7
1999	14,141	$38.6
2000	16,008	$45.2
2001	17,405	$53.7
2002	19,921	$55.7
2003	19,124	$48.9

Note. Data extracted from the Web site of the U.S. Equal Employment Opportunity Commission (www.eeoc.gov/stats/adea.html).
[a]Not including monetary benefits obtained through litigation.

who now make up about half of the workforce, and by 2004 even the youngest of them turned 40 and therefore became covered by federal age-discrimination laws. The oldest workers, who are most likely to face bias, are among the fastest growing part of the workforce. Workers over age 65 increased by 20% in the 1990s; workers over age 75 increased more than 80% from 1980 to 2000.

Precise estimates of the incidence of age discrimination are hard to determine. The EEOC collects data on age discrimination complaints (as seen in Table 2.1), but it is difficult to know for sure whether these numbers reflect an overestimate or an underestimate of real incidence. For example, employees who have been terminated, or applicants who have been turned down for employment, may be eager to attribute such actions to age discrimination rather than personal attributes that might have contributed to the decision. On the other hand, workers or applicants who have been the subject of adverse actions because of their age may either be unaware that they have been discriminated against or unwilling to file a complaint. Faley et al. (1984) have suggested that much of the increase in numbers of age discrimination lawsuits and complaints is attributable to age stereotyping and to ignorance by many organizations and their leaders of the legal rights guaranteed older workers by federal and state laws.

Nonetheless, it is obvious that age continues to work against many older men and women, as evident in the length of time it takes so many to find employment, the wage loss so many experience on reemployment, and the size of awards to victims of discrimination (Rix, 2002). For example, after the Supreme Court ruled in 2000 that individuals could not sue state entities for damages under federal age-bias laws, the EEOC decided to represent 1,700 retired police officers, firefighters, and other safety officers who charged the California Employees Retirement System with discriminating in benefits. Subsequently, the retirement system agreed to pay $250 million—at that time the largest settlement for any kind of discrimination in EEOC history. Similarly, Ford Motor Company is paying more than $10.5 million to settle suits by older managers who claimed that its evaluation system discriminated against them ("Automaker Is Set to Pay $10.5 Million in Suit," 2001). In addition, McDonnell-Douglas is paying $36 million in partial settlement of a suit by about 1,100 older workers who said that the company laid them off to save pension costs and medical benefits (Cohen, 2003).

The Age Discrimination in Employment Act and Related Law

The ADEA is the primary federal statute for dealing with age discrimination complaints. It was passed by Congress and signed into law by President Lyndon Johnson in December 1967. The legislation was designed to protect individuals age 40 and older from employment discrimination on the basis of age and to promote job opportunities for older workers. The ADEA was amended in 1974 to cover government employees and in 1978 to abolish mandatory retirement for federal employees.

Under the ADEA, it is unlawful for an employer to discriminate against a person on the basis of age with respect to any terms, conditions, or privileges of employment. Thus, job assignments, training opportunities, promotions, pay increases, layoffs, retirement, overtime, benefits, vacation, and all other personnel decisions must be made without regard to employee age (Rosen & Jerdee, 1985). The following quote, from the ADEA, provides a good perspective on the thinking of Congress at the time the legislation was enacted.

(a) The Congress hereby finds and declares that—
   (1) in the face of rising productivity and affluence, older workers find themselves disadvantaged in their efforts to retain employment, and especially to regain employment when displaced from jobs;
   (2) the setting of arbitrary age limits regardless of potential for job performance has become a common practice, and certain otherwise desirable practices may work to the disadvantage of older persons;
   (3) the incidence of unemployment, especially long-term unemployment with resultant deterioration of skill, morale, and employer acceptability is, relative to the younger ages, high among older workers; their numbers are great and growing; and their employment problems grave;
   (4) the existence in industries affecting commerce, of arbitrary discrimination in employment because of age, burdens commerce and the free flow of goods in commerce.
(b) It is therefore the purpose of this chapter to promote employment of older persons based on their ability rather than age; to prohibit arbitrary age discrimination in employment; to help employers and workers find ways of meeting problems arising from the impact of age on employment.

The ADEA binds every employer that has 20 or more employees and that is covered by federal labor laws as well as employment agencies, labor organizations, the federal government, and state and local governments. Employment agencies may not classify or refuse to refer individuals on the basis of their age. Labor unions are prohibited from using age to exclude or expel individuals from membership, attempt to or cause an employer to discriminate on the basis of age, or classify or refuse to refer individuals because of age. It does not, however, apply to elected officials or independent contractors (McCann & Giles, 2002).

Every state has its own laws that prohibit age discrimination in employment, and in some states, greater protection is afforded the older worker than can be found in the ADEA. For example, at least 45 states have laws that expand coverage to firms that are too small (i.e., fewer than 20 employees) to be covered by federal labor laws and the ADEA (M. L. Levine, 1988). The ADEA is enforced by state age discrimination agencies in many states and by the EEOC. When individuals believe they have been subjected to age discrimination in violation of the ADEA, they should file charges with their state agency (if their state has one) and with the EEOC. In many states, the EEOC contracts with the state fair employment practice agency to process age discrimination charges.

Exceptions to the Age Discrimination in Employment Act

There are several important exceptions to the ADEA's general prohibitions (ADEA, 2004). All have figured prominently in court cases since the ADEA's enactment, because if an employer can prove that an exception applies, the employer's activities do not violate the ADEA.

First, the law recognizes that age may sometimes be a bona fide occupational qualification (BFOQ) reasonably necessary to the normal operation of the business. When using the defense of BFOQ in an age-discrimination lawsuit, the employer must show that employees over the age of 40 are not capable of performing the job in a manner that is reasonably necessary to the normal operation of the particular business. This BFOQ exception has tended to be useful within a limited scope and application, per EEOC guidelines and court decisions. The courts have given this defense the greatest deference with jobs that involve safety factors (Doering, Rhodes, & Schuster, 1983).

Second, adverse personnel action is allowed if it is based on reasonable factors other than age (RFOA). The employer cannot exclude older workers from a position simply because doing so would be more cost effective. Rather, the employer must establish that an employee was not able to satisfactorily perform a valid job requirement or test. Reasonable factors have ranged from lack of basic job skills to broad, organization-wide problems. For example, when an employer is forced to reduce the workforce for reasons beyond its control (generally economic), the discharge of older employees is considered to be due to RFOA if the reduction is not primarily of older workers. Unlike BFOQ defenses, those based on RFOAs are available only as individual case-by-case exceptions. Defenses most frequently offered by defendants tend to be either related to economic considerations (e.g., reductions-in-force, personnel decisions based directly on employment costs) or noneconomic considerations (e.g., violation of company policy, uncooperativeness, poor performance, lack of training, nearness to retirement; Faley et al., 1984).

The "good cause" exception allows the employer to discharge or discipline an employee, even though he or she is part of a protected class, if it can be shown that age is not a determining factor in the decision. When using this exception as a defense in an age-discrimination suit, the employer must be able to present demonstrable evidence that the employee's performance has fallen below reasonable and clearly articulated organizational standards (Shea, 1991).

The last exception, the seniority system exception, holds that differentiation on the basis of age is allowed where the employer is abiding by the terms of a bona fide seniority system or any bona fide employee benefit plan, such as a retirement, pension, or insurance plan, and these terms are not simply a means of evading the purposes of the act. Although what constitutes "bona fide" varies on the basis of the details of individual cases, several common themes have emerged from court cases. First, courts tend to focus on whether a retirement plan has existed for some time or just prior to an employee's retirement. Second, courts often examine whether the plan pays out a nominal sum or provides more substantial benefits. Third, the courts also tend to examine whether the employer has closely followed the terms of the plan

(Doering et al., 1983). As noted by H. L. Sterns, Doverspike, and Lax (2005), the benefits area is one of the more complex areas of the law and is in the process of evolving to take into account shifts in health care economics and policy.

In general, then, employers may not use the relative costs of hiring, training, or retaining older workers as part of a BFOQ argument. Additionally, employers may not discriminate on the basis of age because of the preferences of their customers or fellow employees. Moreover, a defense may not be based on stereotypical assumptions that disqualify an entire age class. For example, a strenuous job cannot be limited to younger persons because the employer believes that all older workers lack the needed strength. Even if most older persons could not do the job, where it is practical to make decisions individually, each person must be given the opportunity to qualify. An employer may not rule out a strong older person for a job just because most other people of that age would not have the requisite strength. Declaring such practices to be discriminatory is the essence of the ADEA.

Proof of Age Discrimination Under the Age Discrimination in Employment Act

There are two basic ways in which a plaintiff can establish a showing of discrimination: disparate treatment and disparate impact. The *disparate treatment* model requires proof that a certain employee was specifically discriminated against. The *disparate impact* model focuses on establishing that a specific employment practice adversely affects all employees within a certain protected group.

To prove disparate treatment, the plaintiff must show that the discrimination was intentional—that is, show proof of an employer motive to act in ways that lead to less favorable employment consequences for older workers. To establish a case for age discrimination in court, an employee must be able to prove that each of the following is true: that the employee (a) is in the 40 or older age group that is protected by ADEA, (b) was qualified for the position or performing satisfactorily in the position, (c) was adversely affected by an employment action, and (d) received less favorable treatment than a younger worker. Direct or indirect evidence must be offered as proof. Direct evidence may involve documented information that the employee was fired (or not hired) because of age or presentation of statistical evidence showing a pattern of discrimination against older workers. Direct evidence is rarely used, however. The most common method is through indirect or circumstantial evidence. In the absence of direct evidence of discrimination, most courts use a three-stage model of proof (McCann & Giles, 2002), which requires the plaintiff to establish a prima facie case, the employer to offer a defense, and then the plaintiff to present evidence that the employer's defense is only a "pretext" (or excuse) for discrimination.

To prove disparate impact, it is only necessary to show that the employment practice under scrutiny had a differential effect on older workers regardless of the motivation (Shea, 1991). Whereas the employer can defend its policy or practice as a reasonable business necessity, the plaintiff can continue to establish a case by showing that a less discriminatory practice could achieve the same result. The vast majority of age-discrimination suits have used the disparate treatment theory. Although there is a consistency to the ADEA case law when the basis of the suit is the disparate treatment doctrine, much disagreement exists when disparate impact is the cause of the action. These disagreements exist not just about the quantity of evidence necessary to establish a claim but whether a claim of disparate impact is actionable under the ADEA at all (Faley et al., 1984).

The federal appellate courts have been in sharp disagreement as to whether disparate impact may be used to prove age discrimination. In 2002, a case before the Supreme Court seemed likely to resolve the conflict and clarify this issue. In *Adams v. Florida Power* (2002), the question at issue was whether a disparate impact theory of liability can be used by plaintiffs suing for age discrimination under the ADEA of 1967 (ADEA, 2004). However, without giving a reason, the Supreme Court declined to resolve the issue at that time, at least on the basis of the facts presented in *Adams* (Zink, 2002). Finally, in March 2005, the Supreme Court ruled that workers over 40 years of age can sue when an employer's actions have a disparate impact on their age group. However, in the case *Smith v. City of Jackson* (2005), the Court noted that disparate impact suits based on age discrimination should be more limited than are race or sex discrimination cases, suggesting that the ADEA still allows an employer to mount a business necessity defense based on an RFOA exception.

Consequently, it appears that it may still be harder for older workers to win a bias claim than it is for the groups covered by Title VII (Civil Rights Act of 1964, 2003). The Supreme Court has held since 1971 that plaintiffs suing under Title VII do not need to show disparate treatment; it is enough to show that a supposedly neutral policy disproportionately hurts a protected group. When that is shown, the employer has the burden of showing that the challenged policy is necessary for the job. Disparate impact is a powerful tool, because it is often hard for workers to prove intentional discrimination. Many of the biggest race- and sex-discrimination lawsuits may not have been won without it (Cohen, 2003). Nevertheless, even though the disparate-treatment model has typically been used to prove age discrimination, the liabilities of employers who lose ADEA suits tend to be substantially larger (Faley et al., 1984).

As important as the ADEA has been for older individuals, it has by no means eliminated discrimination against them. Moreover, as Rix (2001) noted, some have suggested a weakening of the ADEA in recent years. For example, in a recent case (*Kimel v. Florida Board of Regents*, 2000), the U.S. Supreme Court held that states are protected from ADEA suits by private individuals under the Eleventh Amendment to the U.S. Constitution. This means that public employees in the states do not have the protection of the ADEA. In a second case (*Hazen Paper Co. v. Biggins*, 1993), involving the termination of an employee based on approaching eligibility for a pension, the Supreme Court ruled that there was no violation of the ADEA because the employer's actions were motivated by some factor other than the employee's age, even though the factor was "time until eligibility for pension," which was highly correlated with age. H. L. Sterns et al. (2005) provided an excellent up-to-date overview of ADEA and relevant case law.

Although there is no dramatic evidence that the ADEA has improved older workers' chances of being hired or has eliminated their chances of being targeted during downsizings, it seems reasonable to conclude that without the ADEA, employers would likely be less equitable in their treatment of older workers than they are. Certainly, many workers who are discriminated against never file charges, and many who file charges do not receive favorable judgments. Still, some do, and the judgments against employers can be costly, not only in financial terms, but in terms of public relations and goodwill. As the workforce continues to age, these latter two costs may be ones that employers are increasingly reluctant to incur.

Conclusion

It is beyond question that ageism plays an especially harmful role in the workplace. Older workers face ageist attitudes and age discrimination (McCann & Giles, 2002). Older worker stereotypes are so pervasive that older workers often just accept them as fact and integrate them into their self-concepts; these stereotypes may also affect the judgments and actions of organizational decision makers, as we have shown. Such widely held societal stereotypes are detrimental to individual and organizational productivity, and although legislation can mandate particular organizational policies, it cannot dictate attitudes or behaviors. If managers do not "buy into" the ADEA law and amendments, they are likely to comply only so far as to avoid the potential for lawsuits. Without a commitment to the ADEA and an understanding of the law from a human resources perspective, managers may never truly change their decision making or behavior toward older employees (Dennis, 1988b).

Unfortunately, as Friedan (1993) has suggested, even forward-thinking human resources personnel have traditionally focused more of their attention toward older workers on helping them prepare for and survive retirement. Rix (1990) highlighted one example of a more proactive approach to avoiding ADEA issues. The Grumman Corporation, which has a history of accommodating older workers, uses "age audits" of the workforce as a way to identify and eliminate potential problems before they become lawsuits. In an age audit, the age distribution of an organization's workforce is compared with that of the broader industry or some other comparable regional or local workforce to identify any discrepancies. The expectation is that the percentage of employees of a certain age should be similar to the percentage of workers of the same age in the larger workforce. Large discrepancies should be cause for further examination, and if older workers are underrepresented in the company, reasons for this should be explored.

Age discrimination continues to be pervasive in the American workplace. Strict adherence to the ADEA is necessary to avoid costly lawsuits. However, a commitment to the law is not sufficient. Management must also be committed to the principle behind the law: that each person should be judged on individual merits and provided with equal opportunity to make the best contribution to the workplace and realize his or her aspirations.

Hall and Mirvis (1995) have suggested that workers in middle and later career and life stages represent a relatively underresearched and untapped resource in the U.S. workforce. However, they see a number of barriers to effective use of older workers caused by stereotypes held about older workers. These barriers include, for example, not attending to the human development needs of older workers when doing reengineering and other system changes. Hall and Mirvis suggested that rather than ignoring their development needs during such times, it may be an opportunity to "mobilize" employees through developmental activities.

Another barrier is the perception that it is too costly to invest in the continued learning and development of older employees. Many firms prefer to ignore or "outplace" older workers and spend their development dollars on younger ones, even though the older worker already represents a significant amount of developmental investment and may in fact possess superior experience as well as superior basic skills. Many organizations also believe that the older worker is too inflexible and difficult to train in the modern organization, despite evidence to the contrary. Hall and Mirvis have also suggested that there is a lingering perception that retraining for the older worker would require too much effort for a relatively small group of employees. However, the fact is that workers over age 55 are making up an increasingly larger proportion of the U.S. workforce as the baby boomers continue to age. Thus, it seems clear that no society can simply ignore the developmental needs of this skilled, experienced cohort.

In the future, older workers can look forward to continuing involvement in work for as long as they have the ability to carry out needed activities. Many older adults will be active and healthy and will be able to perform most jobs with great success. Nevertheless, as H. L. Sterns and Huyck (2001) have suggested, they will need to be responsible for their own careers and to be proactive about maintaining and updating their skills to remain competitive. In addition, with continued education and training about aging and work, managers can reduce or avoid age discrimination complaints and lawsuits as well as increase the effective use of their mature workforce. The use of older workers not only can help support the growing and changing goals and objectives of organizations in a global economy, but it can also provide meaningful work roles for middle-aged and older individuals.

3

Physical Capabilities, Cognitive Abilities, and Job Performance

In this chapter we review research on physical and cognitive abilities over the life span of a person, with an emphasis on the nature of declines in these abilities among older adults. Overall, research on aging suggests that physical and cognitive abilities do decline in older age. However, as we discuss in the sections that follow, these declines may not always generalize to deficits in on-the-job performance (e.g., Salthouse, 1990; Salthouse & Maurer, 1996). In fact, older workers generally seem to adapt well and to compensate for declining abilities by adjusting their approach to the job (e.g., the selection, optimization, and compensation model; Baltes & Baltes, 1990b). Furthermore, considerable individual differences exist among people and across abilities and skills. We turn now to a closer look at the available research and its implications for an aging workforce.

Physical Capabilities

Some of our physical and sensory capabilities tend to decline with age. It is important to note, however, that general statements about such decline mask considerable individual variation in physical aging. Physical capabilities are a product of both genetic heritage and environment, and variation in both across persons produces dramatic variation in observed physical and sensory capabilities as the process of aging unfolds (Sheppard & Rix, 1977).

Aging is generally associated with both functional loss and declining homeostasis (McDonald, 1988). *Functional loss* refers to some functions of the body operating at a reduced capacity. These may include muscle strength, aerobic capacity, cardiac function, and sensory perception. We discuss a number of these below. The *decline in homeostasis* refers to the reduced ability of the body to maintain normal operation across environments and a slowing of the process of returning to normal. For example, older persons are more affected by extremes of heat and cold because of their reduced capacity to adjust to temperature changes. They recover more slowly from altered sleep and meal patterns than younger people and thus may develop more intolerance of shift work. They are more susceptible to stress. They are less able to ward off illness, take longer to recover from injury, and are thus more susceptible to disease and chronic health conditions (Hale, 1990; Hansson, DeKoekkoek, Neece, & Patterson, 1997).

A decline in physical strength with age has been well documented (e.g., Rosen & Jerdee, 1985; A. A. Sterns, Sterns, & Hollis, 1996; Warr, 1994). This loss of strength occurs because with age, bones become lighter and more brittle, vertebrae move closer together, and both muscle tone and muscle mass decline. Body composition changes: Lean muscle mass decreases and fat levels increase. With the decline in lean mass, basal metabolic rate drops because the energy required to maintain normal body function drops (McDonald, 1988).

Cardiac and aerobic capacities tend to decline with age (McDonald, 1988). Our lungs lose some of their breathing capacity, the resting heart rate drops, blood pressure increases, cardiac output decreases, and the elasticity of the veins and arteries decreases.

Psychomotor ability also shows declines with age (Forteza & Prieto, 1994). We take longer to react to stimuli, require more time to carry out movements, and show decreased performance at tasks requiring speeded and coordinated response.

Changes in the two most important sensory functions, sight and hearing, occur with age (Forteza & Prieto, 1994). Visual acuity starts to decline between ages 40 and 50, such that we have more difficulty seeing distant objects and require more light to see them. Visual accommodation declines, making it more difficult to focus on close objects. Visual adaptation also declines, making it more difficult to adapt to sudden light changes. As we age, we also experience chromatic distortion that leaves us with reduced sensitivity to colors such as blue and violet. With regard to hearing, we first lose some sensitivity to high-pitched sounds and later to low-pitched ones. We lose some ability to distinguish between concurrent sounds, often observed in increasing difficulty understanding conversations. We find it more difficult to locate the sources of sounds. We also experience more interference from background noise. With regard to other sensory abilities, data are less conclusive. However, Forteza and Prieto (1994) noted that declines in the sense of touch and sense of balance may require job redesign, in part to prevent accidents.

It does not automatically follow that these declines result in lower work performance. First, great individual variation in the aging process means that for a given person, the capability to perform all tasks is not reduced in tandem (Sheppard & Rix, 1977). Second, the declines are very gradual and are not so precipitous that they affect work performance in the majority of jobs. Third, it is possible to compensate for many of these declines through, for example, corrective eyeglasses, change in work strategies, and job redesign. (We return to the topic of job redesign in chap. 7.) As a result of their experience, older persons often move to jobs that are less dependent on physical capacity (Hale, 1990; Warr, 1994). Finally, some of the declines can be slowed through environmental intervention. Wellness programs, for example, can increase functional capacity; Sonnenfeld (1988) cited research showing that regular exercise can "set the clock back 25 to 45 years" (p. 200). Wellness programs can also improve mental outlook, reduce health care costs, and reduce lost work time (Hale, 1990; McDonald, 1988).

Cognitive Abilities

Perhaps the most comprehensive research program on cognitive abilities and aging has been conducted by K. Warner Schaie

(Schaie, 1983, 1993, 1994) in the Seattle Longitudinal Study. Schaie and colleagues have followed several cohorts of adults from age 25 through 88 and beyond. The design of the study has been to test in a laboratory setting a new cohort of adults every 7 years beginning in 1956 and extending through 1998. Starting in 1963 and at each 7-year interval, attempts were also made to test all previously tested cohorts. So in 1963, for example, a new group of 997 persons was tested, but the first cohort was also contacted to return for testing (average age by then being 32 years old), and 303 of the original 500 did in fact participate. In 1970, Schaie and colleagues tested a new cohort of 705, but again, the two earlier cohorts were also represented (Ns = 162 and 420, respectively, with average ages of 39 and 32). Regarding the samples, Schaie (1994) estimated that only the bottom 25% of the socioeconomic range was not represented. Sample members have included crafts and service workers, a variety of professional people, and adults from a reasonably wide range of white- and blue-collar occupations.

The test battery administered has included measures of verbal, spatial, reasoning, numerical, and work fluency abilities. Rigidity–flexibility was also measured in the early years of the study, and beginning with the 1984 cycle, the primary mental abilities of verbal comprehension, verbal memory, spatial orientation, inductive reasoning, numerical ability, and perceptual speed were measured at the latent construct level (i.e., with multiple marker tests), along with measures of self-rated ability declines and health history.

Results of the longitudinal data suggest, first, that except for perceptual speed, which begins declining between ages 25 and 32, all abilities show modest increases from age 25 until about age 46, when they level off or begin to decline slightly. Ability × Gender interactions were also identified, with women performing better in the areas of verbal comprehension and inductive reasoning than men, and men performing better in the areas of spatial orientation and numerical ability than women. Gender differences also occur in ability declines: When abilities are categorized as *fluid* (i.e., abilities in reasoning and related higher mental processes) versus *crystallized* (i.e., abilities related to already acquired knowledge), women decline earlier in fluid ability, men earlier in crystallized ability.

In general, four of the six mental abilities Schaie and colleagues studied reached an asymptote (peaked and then leveled off) in early middle age and then declined modestly after that (Schaie, 1994). As mentioned, perceptual speed began declining by age 25; numerical ability reached an asymptote earlier, with fairly steep declines beginning about age 60. Regarding the older age ranges, comparing ages 25 and 88, there was virtually no decline in verbal ability, with declines of 0.5 standard deviation for inductive reasoning and verbal memory, 1.0 standard deviation for spatial orientation, and 1.5 standard deviations for numerical ability and perceptual speed.

More recent work largely supports these findings for declines in cognitive ability. McArdle, Ferrer-Caja, Hamagami, and Woodcock (2002) found that fluid intelligence declined among older adults whereas crystallized intelligence did not. Similarly, Finkel, Reynolds, McArdle, Gatz, and Pedersen (2003) found across a 6-year period that crystallized intelligence remained stable among older adults, and most other abilities declined linearly. An exception was cognitive abilities with a speed component, which showed accelerating declines after age 65.

In a cross-sectional study relating scores on the General Aptitude Test Battery (Hunter, 1980) and age, Avolio and Waldman (1994) found somewhat greater declines in cognitive abilities with age. Correlations between age and General Aptitude Test Battery subtests were as follows: general intelligence ($r = -.15$); verbal ability ($r = -.10$); numerical ability ($r = -.17$); form perception ($r = -.39$); motor coordination ($r = -.28$); finger dexterity ($r = -.35$); and manual dexterity ($r = -.28$). However, when education and occupation type were controlled for, these correlations were lower. Forteza and Prieto (1994) reviewed age-related changes in sensory, perceptual, psychomotor, and cognitive abilities, and they found on average significant declines in hearing and sight, physical strength and endurance, mental speed, perceptual and spatial abilities, and short-term memory.

Another cognitive-related domain where older adults are assumed to perform more poorly than younger adults is in computer-related tasks. Czaja and Sharit (1993) asked women ages 25 to 70 years to perform three simulated computer-interactive tasks. Results showed that age had a significant impact on task performance, with older women having longer response times and more errors. In a similar study, Czaja and Sharit (1998) had participants from three age groups (20–39, 40–59, and 60–75) perform a computer data-entry task. They found that the oldest group completed significantly less of the task than the other two groups, but after controlling for differences in quantity, they found no age differences in types of errors made. Finally, Salthouse, Hambrick, Lukas, and Dell (1996) asked adults of varying ages to perform several time-management tasks designed to simulate complex work activities. Results of the research indicated large age differences in performance, with more than 70% of the age-related variance consistent with measures of processing speed obtained before the tasks were performed.

Thus, Schaie's work especially demonstrates that on average, most cognitive abilities are at least gradually declining as people reach their late 50s. This is especially true for perceptual speed and numerical ability. The emphasis here, however, should be *on average*; there are large individual differences in when and how much these mental abilities decline among older persons. In fact, Schaie (1994); Warr (1998); and Reynolds, Finkel, Gatz, and Pedersen (2002), among others, have observed that the standard deviations in abilities increase with older study participants.

Factors Associated With Cognitive Ability and Aging

Because of the large individual differences in cognitive abilities among older adults, we might ask: Are there reliable correlates of these differences? The answer appears to be yes, for a number of factors.

A central factor affecting individual functioning in older adults is health, including cardiovascular fitness (e.g., Hertzog, Schaie, & Gribbin, 1978). Barnes, Yaffe, Satariano, and Tager (2003) showed a relationship between cardiovascular fitness in older adults ages 59 to 88 and declines in all cognitive abilities tested 6 years later, especially global cognitive functioning. The direction of causation has not been well established, and it is possible that lifestyle variables lead to both the onset of such diseases and intellectual decline (Schaie, 1994).

A second factor seems to be involvement in complex, intellectually stimulating activities, such as a job requiring considerable intellectual activity. These kinds of activities are associated with lower rates of decline in older workers. For example, Masunaga and Horn (2001) found that older people with high levels of expertise on a complex job showed very little decline in deductive and fluid reasoning, short-term memory, and cognitive speed. Morrow, Leirer, Altiteri, and Fitzsimmons (1994) studied pilots and age-matched nonpilots on an air traffic control task and a cognitive task unrelated to this domain. Results showed that relevant expertise eliminated age differences in the air traffic task but that age-related differences were significant for pilots and nonpilots on the domain irrelevant task. Finally, Bosma, van Boxtel, Ponds, Houx, and Jolles (2003), using data from the Maastricht Aging Study (Jolles, van Boxtel, Ponds, Metsemakers, & Houx, 1998), found that seniors with higher educational level showed less decline in information processing speed and general cognitive functioning than their less educated counterparts. It is important to note that these differences were lower when the lower education group had relatively high levels of work-related mental challenge.

Leisure activities like reading and participation in continuing education also can contribute to the maintenance of cognitive abilities (Gribbin, Schaie, & Parham, 1980). In fact, Bosma et al. (2002) found that participation in mental, social, and physical activities mitigated the decline in cognitive ability over a 3-year period. Similarly, Schaie (1983) suggested that older adults who have a more "engaged" lifestyle are more likely to maintain levels of cognitive functioning. Some support for this position was provided by Arbuckle, Gold, and Andres (1986), who found that older people whose involvement in intellectually stimulating activities was minimal had lower levels of intellectual performance. It is interesting that in the Bosma et al. (2002) study, seniors with relatively high levels of cognitive ability at initial testing were more likely to increase the amount of these activities, suggesting a reciprocal relationship between cognitive ability and participation in such activities.

A related factor is having a history of involvement in intellectually stimulating activities and, even more broadly, a history of living in a favorable environment, including having been well educated and having had access to money (Gribbin et al., 1980). Yet another correlate of avoiding cognitive decline as an older adult is living with someone (especially a spouse) who has a high level of cognitive functioning (e.g., Gruber & Schaie, 1986). Finally, possessing a flexible personal style into older age (Schaie, 1984) and maintaining relatively high levels of cognitive processing speed (Schaie, 1989; Zimfrich, 2002) are both associated with maintenance of cognitive abilities as a senior.

The question might also be asked: Are declines in abilities among older people reversible? That is, can training improve seniors' abilities? This and related questions have been addressed as part of Schaie and colleagues' research program. In particular, Schaie and Willis (1986) and Willis and Schaie (1986) focused on educational interventions related to spatial orientation and inductive reasoning. For the sample, they identified people 65 years of age or older and who scored low in the last two testing periods (a total of 14 years) in one or both of these abilities. Between 179 and 228 individuals participated in the studies.

The initial training intervention consisted of five 1-hour sessions for each of the abilities. The design was pretest–intervention–posttest, with each training group (i.e., spatial orientation or inductive reasoning) serving as the control for the other group. Results showed that about two thirds of participants significantly improved after the interventions, and 40% actually improved to levels attained before the 14-year decline. Similarly, Baltes, Dittman-Kohli, and Kliegl (1986) showed that relatively brief training programs can improve cognitive ability in both the areas of fluid and crystallized intelligence for older adults at least to age 80. These findings are encouraging and suggest that engaging in activities related to an ability helps to maintain that ability or at least slow its decline.

Methodological Observations

A few methodological observations should be made about research comparing the cognitive abilities of persons at different times in their life spans. First, longitudinal studies are almost always better than cross-sectional studies. This is primarily because of potential cohort effects that confound age differences in cross-sectional research. The best way to estimate these cohort effects is to test multiple cohorts at the same ages and examine mean differences in test scores for the different cohorts. The Seattle Longitudinal Study did just that for cohorts born around 1900 all the way to 1966, testing them every 7 years.

Results show large cohort differences for many of the abilities examined in the study. For example, inductive reasoning and verbal memory increased nearly linearly by 1.5 standard deviations from the earliest to the latest cohort (averaging across all of the testing periods for each cohort). Another pattern was increases in average ability for the early cohorts, followed by a leveling in the middle cohorts, and then a decline in the latest cohorts. This was noted for numerical ability, perceptual speed, and verbal ability. Substantive reasons for these differences are unclear except that the improving abilities may be a function of increasing educational levels and better nutrition in later cohorts. However, the main point here is a methodological one. Increasing levels of an ability mean that in cross-sectional research, decline in the ability with age are underestimated. More generally, any cohort differences render across-age comparisons inaccurate.

A second methodological observation is that even longitudinal studies have a potential problem interpreting across-age ability levels, especially as the sample members reach advanced age. This is because as the cohort being followed reaches older age, those who drop out of the sample may have done so because of dementia or even death. In fact, the Scottish Mental Survey results provide a rather direct estimate of this bias. In 1932 and again in 1947, practically every 11-year-old in school in Scotland was tested ($Ns = 89,498$ and $70,805$) using the Morey House Tests (Scottish Council for Research in Education, 1933). These tests, although not directly measuring general cognitive ability, were shown to correlate .80 with a commonly used test of cognitive ability, the Stanford–Binet (Deary, Whiteman, Starr, Whalley, & Fox, 2004). The 1932 and 1947 cohorts were followed up to identify deaths and various debilitating illnesses among cohort members. Using psychometric cognitive ability at age 11 as the independent variable, differences were tested between those deceased and those alive at age 76.

Large differences were found, with higher ability being associated with considerably lower mortality rates (Whalley & Deary, 2001). Similarly, higher ability was associated with lower levels of cancer, cardiovascular disease, and hospital stays (Deary, Whalley, & Starr, 2003). Thus, longitudinal studies may on balance underestimate average declines in ability because the more able members of the cohort are likely to remain in the sample.

Job Performance

Although the consensus is that adults older than about age 55 show declines in several abilities, research correlating age with job performance generally finds almost no correlation between the two. For example, in an early review, Rhodes (1983) concluded that there was evidence for at least four different age–job performance relations: weak positive, weak negative, an inverted U, and nonsignificant. In their meta-analysis investigating this relationship, McEvoy and Cascio (1989) found a correlation of .06 between age and job performance. Waldman and Avolio (1986) also conducted a meta-analysis and found an overall mean correlation of near zero between age and job performance, but they also identified a moderator of this relationship. When performance measures were objective, the relation was positive; when ratings were used as the performance measure, the mean correlation was negative (see also H. L. Sterns & Alexander, 1987). The authors noted that one possible reason for the latter finding is rater bias against older workers.

Another moderator that has been studied is job type. Waldman and Avolio (1986) found a more positive correlation between age and job performance for professional jobs compared with nonprofessional jobs. McEvoy and Cascio (1989) did not find this moderator; however, Warr (1994) and Beehr and Bowling (2002) suggested searching for moderators among job characteristics that might relate to age (e.g., jobs where experience is related to job performance or jobs that require certain abilities that are known to decline with age).

Yet another potential moderator is the dimension of job performance. For example, Gilbert, Collins, and Valenzi (1993) examined performance ratings on different dimensions for workers ages 25 to over 50. For the dimensions technical competence, overall performance, and job commitment, the highest ratings were associated with 25- to 30-year-olds; the lowest ratings were given to those over 50. For the dimension of work relations, the pattern was the opposite, with workers over age 50 receiving the highest performance ratings. On the other hand, Schappe (1998) and Williams and Shaw (1999) found virtually no correlation between age and citizenship performance.

Although not exactly a dimension of job performance, another dependent variable studied in relation to age is on-the-job injuries or accidents. The incidence of injuries is actually lower for older workers (e.g., H. L. Sterns, Barrett, & Alexander, 1985); however, once injured, they generally take longer to heal and get back to work. In Australia, for example, Thomas, Browning, and Greenwood (1994) found there was a strong relation between age and long-term compensation awards involving disabilities. The inference is that although accidents and injuries on the job are fewer for older workers, when they do occur older workers are likely to require more time before they return to the job.

Other researchers have drawn conclusions about the perceptions people have of older workers. They are perceived to be harder to train, less able to deal with technology, more accident prone, and less motivated (Rosen & Jerdee, 1976; Stagner, 1985), but they are perceived as dependable, cooperative, conscientious, consistent, and knowledgeable (Rosen & Jerdee, 1976).

It is interesting to speculate about the reasons for the low correlation between age and job performance. Several explanations have been offered. Park (1994) suggested that older workers often have jobs they are very familiar with and often have considerable practice and experience with their job tasks, thus allowing for successful performance even if broader cognitive functioning declines. Moreover, older workers may have developed complex detailed knowledge structures (i.e., expertise) that compensate for any loss in general skills or abilities. An example of this was provided in a study by Salthouse (1984), who found that the reaction time of typists declined with age, but their typing speed was the same as their younger counterparts because older typists tend to read ahead farther, thus readying themselves for entering that material. Finally, senior workers may often have more access to coworker support to help them with their tasks.

Schooler, Caplan, and Oates (1998) suggested the following reasons for smaller or no age differences in job performance compared with the age differences in cognitive abilities found in laboratory settings: (a) Expertise and experience may help make up for declines in cognitive functioning; (b) lab tasks tend to push people to their cognitive limits, whereas actual jobs usually do not; (c) older people with large declines in cognitive abilities have often left the workplace; and (d) older workers are more motivated and satisfied with their jobs and thus tend to try harder.

Older workers can compensate for overall deficits in other ways as well. Landy (*Mandatory Retirement*, 1996) conducted a congressionally mandated study regarding the effects of age on the effectiveness of public service workers. One important finding was that job experience and, especially, physical fitness could reduce the effects of age on health and safety problems among older patrol officers and firefighters. For older firefighters, aerobic capacity is typically lower (e.g., Sothmann, Saupe, Jasenof, & Blaney, 1992), but exercise and overall physical fitness can reduce the gap between older and younger firefighters.

The notion of older workers compensating for certain cognitive and physical deficits leads to a related issue, the effects of job and organization change on older workers and how this change might be managed to help ensure more productivity for these workers. In particular, a trend that has been evident in organizations is movement away from workers mastering a small number of tasks and continuing to work on those tasks. Instead, organization members often work in teams or on task forces that involve more variety in tasks and assignments. This kind of work environment can require adaptability and lead to increased stress; furthermore, these features may not be compatible with older workers' needs, preferences, or personal characteristics.

Some have offered ideas for reducing the problems older workers may face with this kind of environment or, more broadly, with job changes in general (e.g., job redesign), to delay their loss to retirement. The most obvious is for employers to consult with workers during any job redesign process. Getting their input has been shown to decrease the stress of the change and increase chances that the older worker decides to remain on the job (Mondy, Sharplin, & Flippo, 1988; Shonk, 1992). Two additional approaches that seem to be useful during job changes are, first, to provide flexibility for the worker (e.g., 4-day work week, telecommuting, or other accommodations), and, second, to provide financial incentives (e.g., more pay or bonuses for taking on more responsibilities; Fyock, 1990; Rosen & Jerdee, 1985).

In addition, relevant training and education can help older employees with their perceptions about the job redesign efforts (Abraham & Hansson, 1995). This approach appears to work best when they are allowed to learn at their own pace and be trained with other more senior employees (Knowles, 1987; Shea, 1991).

Finally, management and coworker support during the change can help. Older workers often need others to understand their special needs and difficulties. In fact, training courses for managers to increase their understanding of these needs have been successful (Dennis, 1988a; Shonk, 1992). Similarly, coworker support has been shown to be important during the job change process, particularly when the redesign effort moves the work environment more toward a team approach (Kouzes & Posner, 1987; LaRocco, House, & French, 1980).

Organizational personnel policies can also be influential in helping or hindering an older worker's reaction to job redesign and change. Two extreme models have been described: the *depreciation model* that views older workers as increasingly less valuable and dispensable, at least toward the end of their work career, and the *conservation model* that treats older employees as valuable human resources worthy of receiving continued training and positive support from management (DeViney & O'Rand, 1988; Hayward, Hardy, & Grady, 1989).

Conclusion

On balance, older workers often perform on jobs as effectively as their younger counterparts. This is especially true when they (a) avoid suffering the physical and cognitive declines usually evident in their age cohort; (b) have a relatively high degree of experience and expertise in their job; (c) have some flexibility in how to approach and accomplish their job; (d) retain a high motivation to succeed on the job; (e) have a job that does not involve a lot of change; (f) receive management and coworker support at work; and (g) get the appropriate job training in an environment that meets the special needs of older workers.

4

Age, Attitudes, Personality, and Successful Aging

In the preceding chapter, we dealt with the effects of aging—both basic physiological and cognitive functioning—on job performance. Apparently, however, being successful in work and nonwork situations is a function not only of an individual's knowledge, skills, and abilities, but also of certain noncognitive attributes. Therefore, in this chapter we discuss (a) relationships between age and job satisfaction, job involvement, and organizational commitment; (b) the role of personality in older people and, indeed, across the entire adult life span; and (c) various coping strategies older workers might use to ensure personal and occupational well-being. We begin with a review of age–job attitude relationships.

Age–Job Attitude Relationships

In cross-sectional studies, there appears to be a small positive correlation between chronological age and job satisfaction. Whereas Warr (1994) estimated the relationship to be relatively modest (between .10 and .20), others have posited a more complex relationship, with job satisfaction relatively high very early in a career (e.g., early 20s), lower between the mid-20s to early 30s, and then rising through the 40s and beyond (see Warr, 1994). If this is the case, the age–job satisfaction relation for individuals in their early 30s and beyond is likely to be stronger than it is for those in their 20s. Kacmar and Ferris (1989) made the excellent methodological point that studies of the age–job satisfaction correlation should control for tenure. In their study, they controlled for organizational tenure, job tenure, and tenure working with present supervisor. They also examined multiple facets of job satisfaction, using the Job Descriptive Index (a multifaceted measure of job satisfaction; Smith, Kendall, & Hulin, 1969). Results showed that for four of the five facets (Supervision, Coworkers, Pay, and Promotions), a U-shaped relationship emerged; with the Work Itself facet, the correlation was positive and linear. So this well-controlled study reported results reasonably similar to the more complex relationship suggested earlier.

There are several possible explanations for this changing relationship across different age groups. First is the model of workers moving from job to job until they find one they like and then staying in that job. One way to test at least partially for this is to control for job level. This kind of analysis, however, generally does not reduce the age–job satisfaction correlation (Birdi, Warr, & Oswald, 1995; Clark & Oswald, 1996).

A second possible explanation for this relationship is cohort differences in levels of job satisfaction. This argument is that cohorts of older workers have always been more satisfied with their jobs, even when they were younger. The argument against this explanation is that average job satisfaction levels over time suggest that job satisfaction is actually reasonably high for some of the younger cohorts as well (Warr, 1998).

A third explanation is that as employees become older, their expectations about what a job should offer are reduced (e.g., Brandstädter & Rothermund, 1994). A fourth is that broader mental health, which may on average be higher for older workers, "causes" the higher levels of job satisfaction (Warr, 1998). However, when life satisfaction, at least as indexed by the admittedly somewhat superficial variables of marital status and number of dependents, is controlled for, the age–job satisfaction relationship is not affected. Clearly, more research is needed on this explanation.

The last potential explanation for the age–satisfaction relationship is the same as with earlier discussions about the age–job performance relationship. That is, older people who had low levels of job satisfaction may have already left the workforce. It is certainly the case that a significantly larger percentage of older people are not working, typically through retirement, than younger people (e.g., Ellison, Melville, & Gutman, 1996). To the extent that older persons who leave the workforce are those less satisfied with their jobs—a plausible hypothesis—the positive relationship between age and job satisfaction tends to be overestimated. On balance, each of these explanations likely has some merit. However, in each case the empirical evidence is somewhat mixed, and it is not clear to what extent the relative contribution to the age–job satisfaction correlation is related to each of these explanations (Warr, 1998).

It appears also that older workers tend to report higher levels of job involvement and organizational commitment (Warr, 1994). Explanations for these relationships may partially parallel the explanations just discussed in connection with job satisfaction, especially the birth cohort effect rationale. The cohorts of older workers are typically more imbued with the Protestant work ethic (Schooler, Caplan, & Oates, 1998), and this could account for higher levels of job involvement and organizational commitment. Another possible explanation is that job autonomy and organizational rewards tend to be higher on average for older workers, and this could in turn account for higher involvement and commitment (Schooler et al., 1998).

Two organizational outcome variables often related to job satisfaction and involvement, as well as organizational commitment, are turnover and absenteeism (Borman, 1991). These variables have also been studied in relation to age. Research suggests a negative correlation between age and turnover, in the range of −.20 to −.25 (e.g., Beehr & Bowling, 2002). Warr (1994) offered two possible explanations for this relationship. First, older workers stay in their jobs because they do not believe other employers are likely to hire someone at their career stage. And second, older workers are likely to be more satisfied because they occupy relatively high-paying jobs and thus tend not to seek employment elsewhere. A "sunk costs model" (i.e., the notion held by the worker that much time and effort have already been expended on this job) has also been suggested as a reason for lower turnover among older employees (Arkes & Blumer, 1985).

A similar negative correlation is found between age and avoidable absences (i.e., absences under the employee's control; Rhodes, 1983; Thompson, Griffiths, & Davison, 2000). However, for unavoidable absences, the correlation with age is positive, presumably because older workers are more likely than younger workers to have health problems that result in absences.

Overall, the picture for job attitudes and related outcomes, as it concerns the older worker, is quite positive for both employers and employees. Older employees are on average more satisfied, show greater commitment and involvement with their jobs and the organization, and tend to stay with the organization longer than younger workers. From a management perspective, older employees are likely to be easier to manage. The stereotype of the cranky old person at work is not supported by the research. These results are also favorable for older workers themselves. There is some evidence that employees can look forward to relatively satisfying work experiences toward the end of their career. The cross-sectional nature of most research in this area renders the conclusion somewhat tentative but certainly suggestive. We now turn to a discussion of the relationship between age and personality.

Age and Personality

A central question related to personality and age is, how coherent and consistent is personality across time? Reportedly, when Jack Block, the renowned personality researcher (see Block, 1971), was asked this question about whether people change in personality over time, he replied that some do and others do not (Ryff, Kwan, & Singer, 2001). Though rather terse, this statement turns out to be reasonably accurate.

An important aspect of any close examination of this age–personality question is the analytical techniques used. Most researchers on personality changes over time use correlational analysis to compare trait scores at different points in time or examine mean trait differences over time by using a repeated measures analysis of variance (ANOVA) statistical technique. High correlations for the correlational approach indicate little change in the rank order of people on that trait. It turns out that research using this strategy shows reasonably high correlations, indicating considerable consistency across the life span, especially in adulthood (e.g., Block, 1971; Costa & McCrae, 1980; Moss & Susman, 1980). The ANOVA approach examines group mean differences in scores on a trait at different times. Researchers using the ANOVA technique tend to find only small changes in adult personality, indicating stability in these scores over time (e.g., Haan, Milsap, & Hartka, 1986).

This research that examines the stability of personality over time has been useful and informative. However, there are certain limitations with these two methods. Correlational analysis ignores possible shifts in mean levels across time. ANOVA results that find no differences could reflect either no change for everyone in the sample or different patterns of change for individuals in the sample, with these changes essentially canceling each other out and thus resulting in small mean differences (but considerable change for individuals). Recent advances in statistical theory and computing have enabled researchers to address some of these issues. We now review four recent studies that used methods more conducive to focusing on change in personality and on the nature of those changes.

An important study was conducted by Helson, Jones, and Kwan (2002) using the California Psychological Inventory (CPI; Gough, 1996) and a sophisticated analytical technique known as hierarchical linear modeling (HLM). This study examined three longitudinal samples tested as many as five times between ages 21 and 75. HLM allows the researcher to separate individual and group effects as well as to examine relationships other than linear, or straight-line, relationships between variables (Bryk & Raudenbush, 1987). HLM allowed Helson et al. to identify nonlinear changes in personality over time for the entire group and for individuals in the samples. That is, with HLM, both the extent and direction of change can be estimated for the group and each person.

Helson et al. (2002) found that for both men and women, there were increases with age in several norm-adherence dimensions (e.g., self-control). They also found decreases over time for all of the social vitality dimensions of the CPI (e.g., Sociability and Social Presence). Finally, their results, along with earlier cross-sectional studies, suggest that personality changes with age are very similar across culture, cohort, and gender. The HLM results gave evidence in several cases of nonlinear change patterns. These findings cast some doubt on the maturational hypothesis (McCrae et al., 1999, 2000), which posits that the vast majority of personality changes occur before age 30, with considerable stability after that. There are two reasons the Helson et al. results run counter to this hypothesis. There is evidence that personality changes occur throughout the life span for most of the traits, with for the most part curvilinear trajectories.

There is also impressive evidence for environmental, event-related change in personality. For example, there is a curvilinear change in dominance and independence, with peaks in middle age when most people in the sample attained their maximum power and status at work. Thus, work experiences and the work-related environment do influence this personality change. Also suggestive are the curvilinear results for responsibility, with a temporary drop for both cohorts from approximately 1960 to 1980, even though the cohorts were born almost 20 years apart. A plausible explanation for this is that this period witnessed the height of individualism, with an emphasis on private and interpersonal experience and a de-emphasis on formal roles and social commitments. Apparently cultural or environmental events do affect personality change.

Cross-sectional studies of personality over the life span are problematic because of possible birth cohort effects. For example, cohorts of older people may be more conscientious because they underwent stricter child rearing practices rather than because of any maturational changes (i.e., they could have been more conscientious throughout their lives than younger people). McCrae et al. (1999) analyzed personality data from five countries other than the United States (Germany, Italy, Portugal, Croatia, and South Korea; total $N = 7,363$) that addressed this problem to some extent. McCrae et al. reasoned that if similar age differences in personality could be demonstrated across five countries, then the differences could not reasonably be attributed to birth cohort effects. This is because to a large extent the historical experiences of the five societies represented in this sample were substantially different.

The McCrae et al. (1999) study was designed to explore cross-sectional similarities and differences in personality across the life span and potentially to address problems with previous cross-sectional research on personality and aging. The authors used data from a single inventory, the revised NEO–FFI Personality Inventory (Costa & McCrae, 1985), to ensure comparability across the national samples. The NEO–FFI measures personality across five broad dimensions or domains. These dimensions are labeled Neuroticism, Extraversion, Conscientiousness, Agreeableness, and Openness to Experience, and because of their relatively wide acceptance in personality research, they are often referred to as "the Big Five" (L. R. Goldberg, 1990, 1993). There are also finer grained subdimensions, or facet scales (30 in all), that are grouped under each of the Big Five dimensions. Male and female participants in the sample were divided into four age groups: 18–21, 22–29, 30–49, and 50 and older.

Results showed that at the Big Five level, the youngest group scored significantly higher than the two oldest groups on neuroticism, extraversion, and openness to experience and significantly lower in agreeableness and conscientiousness. At the facet level, the age differences within the neuroticism dimension were largely due to differences in the impulsiveness facet. Differences were much smaller for the anxiety and depression facets. Within extraversion, the excitement-seeking and positive emotions facets created the largest age differences, with warmth, assertiveness, and activity less responsible for those differences. Within the openness to experience and agreeableness dimensions, all of the facets showed modest differences. Finally, for conscientiousness, the dutifulness facet showed the largest differences. In general, then, across the 30 facets older men and women seem to be better at impulse control, more responsible, and lower in thrill seeking.

In addition, differences in these age patterns for the five countries were small. That is, differences in personality between younger and older adults were very similar across all five countries. The authors suggested that not only is personality genetically determined to a significant extent (e.g., McGue, Bouchard, Iacono, & Lykken, 1993; Riemann, Angleitner, & Strelau, 1997), but it may be that genetics play a role in determining maturational changes as well.

As mentioned, the finding of similar change patterns across cultures also speaks to interpretation problems with previous cross-sectional data on personality and aging. The birth cohort explanation for those results is less plausible according to this study. As McCrae et al. (1999) put it, "Respondents who grew up during the totalitarian regimes of Hitler, Mussolini, and Salazar showed the same personality profiles relative to their children as Americans who grew up in the era of Franklin Roosevelt" (p. 474).

Jones and Meredith (1996) conducted longitudinal research on stability and change in personality over a 30- to 40-year period. Like Helson et al. (2002), they were most interested in exploring personality change over time. They used a complex analytical technique known as *latent curve analysis*, a method that allows a view of individuals' unique patterns of change over time (Meredith & Tisak, 1990). It is similar to HLM but has more flexibility. Personality data were available for a sample of approximately 100–200 men and women tested at intervals of about 10 years from age 20 through age 60. The target personality variables were self-confidence, assertiveness, cognitive commitment (e.g., values intellect, is introspective), outgoingness, dependability, and warmth.

Most people gained in self-confidence between ages 30 and 50, leveling off after age 50. Assertiveness showed considerable consistency, with men scoring higher across the entire life span. Cognitive commitment increased from 18 to 30, remained steady from 30 to 50, and then decreased somewhat from age 50 to 60. The main finding for outgoingness was that women showed consistently higher scores and that both men and women increased their scores over time. Dependability showed an increase from age 18 to 30 and then stabilized across the rest of the life span. For warmth, the individual differences in across-time trajectories varied so greatly that no group pattern could be determined.

In addition, analyses with the latent curve method indicated individual differences in the extent and direction of change over time. For example, regarding self-confidence, for one of the two cohort groups studied, 32% significantly increased, 2% significantly decreased, and 66% remained the same across the life span studied. Overall, the results suggest adult developmental effects in self-confidence, cognitive commitment, outgoingness, and dependability. Assertiveness appears more consistent across time.

Finally, the merit of examining individual differences with the latent curve strategy was convincingly demonstrated. Most notably with warmth, a more traditional analytic method of analysis (ANOVA) would likely have shown little change longitudinally; this would have been highly misleading, masking the wide variation in trajectories for individuals in the sample.

An intriguing basic question about personality and work is, do the job and the workplace bring about change in personality, or is the effect in the opposite direction, with personality leading to choices of jobs and work settings? One theoretical framework, the attraction–selection–attrition formulation proposed by Schneider (e.g., Schneider, Smith, Taylor, & Fleenor, 1998), suggests the latter. People gravitate to jobs and organizations that fit with their values, interests, and personalities, and provided the fit is good, they tend to stay in those jobs and organizations. There is some evidence for the validity of the attraction–selection–attrition model (Schneider et al., 1998; Schneider, Goldstein, & Smith, 1995).

However, recently some evidence emerged for the former possibility. Roberts, Caspi, and Moffitt (2003) studied a sample of 18-year-olds, relatively new in the workforce, and then tracked this group for the next 8 years, conducting a second data gathering when they were age 26. A personality inventory was administered at Time 1 and then again at Time 2. In addition, each person's work experiences, such as the complexity of their job, their work involvement and satisfaction, and their feelings about financial security were measured. Roberts et al. adopted a "sociogenic" perspective (Inkeles & Levinson, 1963), which posits that social structure shapes personality functioning; in this context work experiences affect change in personality. The authors found that work experiences during their early career years (ages 18–26) were associated with personality changes. Furthermore, the traits that had a role in selecting members of the sample into the organization at Time 1 tended to be the traits that showed the most positive change across the 8 years. An interpretation of this finding is that work experiences will deepen and elaborate traits we already have rather than bring out traits that are not as evident in us.

The implication of these results for older workers is that the effects of work experiences on personality are likely to be even larger because of their considerably longer time in the workforce compared to this sample. Accordingly, although there is considerable coherence and stability in personality across older persons' lives, there are predictable changes in personality as well, and as suggested by this study, some of those changes are likely a result of cumulative work experience.

Thus, although cross-sectional data must be interpreted with caution, these studies have recently provided some useful findings. For example, Siu, Spector, Cooper, and Donald (2001) studied three samples of Hong Kong managers and found that older managers reported fewer sources of stress, better coping, and a more internal locus of control (i.e., they felt more control over their work environment) than their younger counterparts. Ones and Viswesvaran (1998) found very small differences between "over age 40" and "under age 40" job applicants (Ns = 724 and 806) on integrity test scores. Warr, Miles, and Platts (2001), also working with large samples, found that older people in the United Kingdom were more conscientious, traditional, and careful in interactions with others, and less sociable, outgoing, change oriented, and career motivated than younger people. These results are similar to some of those discussed previously (e.g., Helson et al., 2002; McCrae et al., 1999).

Erikson's (1959) concept of generativity in developmental theory suggests that during midlife individuals typically move beyond concerns about the self and identity and the interpersonal focus on intimacy to concerns for others, including family and younger colleagues. The generativity concept has received attention again recently (McAdams & de St. Aubin, 1998). An interesting feature about generativity is that it falls outside of the usual trait domain (e.g., the Big Five or the CPI dimensions). Thus, although there is considerable evidence for stability and coherence in many of the typically targeted personality constructs, change is more evident from this developmental perspective.

In summary, although there is considerable evidence for stability of personality, particularly during the adult life span, recent research has found reliable shifts in some traits for certain periods of life. Evidence has also emerged for substantial individual differences in trajectories on several traits, with increases, decreases, and stability evident for different people.

First, at the Big Five level, Neuroticism, Extraversion, and Openness to Experience tend to decline with age, and Agreeableness and Conscientiousness have upward trajectories across the adult life span. Declines in Neuroticism derive primarily from reduced impulsiveness later in life. Likewise, increases in Conscientiousness seem largely a result of increased self-control, dutifulness, and other norm-adherence-related constructs. Regarding Extraversion, the declines with age seem primarily due to reduced social vitality, including lower sociability, social presence, and excitement seeking. For Agreeableness, there appear to be gradual increases across the life span, including modestly higher standing on trust, straightforwardness, and compliance. Finally, lower scores for older adults on Openness seem to be associated with lower behavioral flexibility. The Openness declines probably tie in with the cognitive literature that shows deficits in speed-related abilities and fluid intelligence (e.g., Schaie, 1994).

With the possible exception of the Openness findings, the personality change results support the hiring of older workers, because they are likely to be less impulsive and more conscientious in carrying out their tasks. The higher level of Agreeableness also means they should get along more smoothly with supervisors, coworkers, and customers, compared with younger workers. From a management perspective, this is highly desirable. Dependability and to a lesser extent agreeableness have been linked to organizational citizenship (e.g., Organ, 1997) or citizenship performance (Borman & Motowidlo, 1993; Borman, Penner, Allen, & Motowidlo, 2001). Citizenship performance has in turn been found to relate to individuals' overall performance and, more broadly, to organizational effectiveness. Thus, it appears that personality characteristics likely to be on average higher for older workers are correlated with positive individual and organizational performance outcomes.

To reinforce this point, Conscientiousness has been found, consistently across all types of occupations and criteria, to be a good predictor of overall good performance (Barrick, Mount, & Judge, 2001). Moreover, Emotional Stability (the inverse of Neuroticism) predicts overall job performance and some specific criteria (e.g., teamwork). Finally, Agreeableness was found to predict teamwork-related criteria (Barrick et al., 2001). These relationships are also favorable for older workers. For all three of these Big Five personality traits, older workers score higher than younger workers.

Another important result is that salient environmental influences associated with the job or with cultural events may cause personality changes. Roberts et al. (2003) showed that work experiences were associated with personality changes, especially those traits important for the hiring decision in the first place. Thus, traits that were useful for successful job performance actually had a positive change trajectory. Moreover, certain important societal effects such as the women's movement (Roberts, Helson, & Klohnen, 2002) and the individualism phenomenon (Helson et al., 2002) appeared to have at least temporarily affected adult personality patterns.

Successful Aging and Quality of Life Issues

The research and discussions about "successful aging" and quality of life have considerable overlap with issues of personality. A very rich and useful formulation of the domain of successful psychological functioning in older age is provided by Ryff (1989). She identified six critical dimensions of positive psychological functioning: (a) self-acceptance—feeling good about oneself and about one's past life; (b) positive relations with others—having high-quality, caring relationships with others; (c) environmental mastery—being able to create an environment in which one can function successfully; (d) autonomy—having the capacity to think and act on one's own, when appropriate; (e) purpose in life—having substantial reasons for living; and (f) personal growth—continuing to strive for personal improvement and development. Ryff and her colleagues have studied the age trajectories of adults on these six dimensions, in both cross-sectional and longitudinal research (e.g., Ryff & Keyes, 1995; Kling, Seltzer, & Ryff, 1997). Across the life stages of young adulthood, midlife, and older age, self-acceptance and positive relations with others show little change. Environmental mastery and autonomy improve with age, and purpose in life and personal growth consistently show declines.

Diehl, Coyle, and Labouvie-Vief (1996) studied coping and defense strategies used by younger and older adults. They found that older persons used strategies of greater impulse control and self-awareness and of lesser aggression than did younger persons. Another area related to the expression of personality involves "life tasks" and setting and maintaining goals. These activities appear to be important for successful aging. For example, Harlow and Cantor (1996) found that participating in social and community service activities was associated with life satisfaction, even after controlling for health and social support. The key to maintaining life satisfaction in older age seems to be flexibility and accommodation in setting and pursuing goals (Ryff et al., 2001). That is, rather than doggedly striving to attain a certain outcome, older persons should pursue goals with some flexibility built in so that if constraints related to old age become an impediment to reaching goals, adjustments can be made to avoid failures.

Similarly, Brandstädter, Wentura, and Rothermund (1999) made the distinction between tenacious goal pursuit and flexible goal adjustment, with the latter being much more appropriate for older people. With this perspective, the path to successful aging and such outcomes as life satisfaction and avoidance of frustration and project failures is to set and pursue goals, but with a willingness to make adjustments and accommodations along the way. A related perspective is that in old age, an increasingly important process is goal choice and the regulation of those choices (Heckhausen & Schultz, 1999). For example, Freund and Baltes (1998) found that flexible goal and life choices were associated with life satisfaction, positive emotions, and absence of loneliness.

Another personality-related variable that appears to be important for understanding successful aging is the resilience construct. Resilience relates to maintaining a high degree of well-being despite setbacks or adversity. This is especially relevant for older people because they typically face a relatively large number of challenges. As part of a 40-year longitudinal study, Singer and Ryff (1999) studied long-term economic adversity and found that this antecedent together with poor or nonexistent close social ties were correlated with *allostatic load* (an index of the degradation of various physiological systems). Allostatic load is in turn associated with health problems and cognitive declines. Note that when older persons have close social and interpersonal relations, these negative outcomes often are avoided (Ryff et al., 2001). Thus, these types of relationships appear important for resilience in older people.

Some of the research reviewed in this section gives hope to older adults. Ryff and colleagues showed that there is improvement, on average, for older people in two of the six factors they described as important for life success: (a) being able to create a functional environment for oneself and (b) having the capacity to be autonomous when appropriate. The purpose in life and personal growth factors unfortunately appear to decline for older persons (Ryff & Keyes, 1995). Two primary strategies for successful aging seem to be (a) setting and maintaining flexible goals that may be adjusted to accommodate any age-related declines in health or mental functioning (Ryff et al., 2001); and (b) participating in social and community activities and maintaining close interpersonal relationships, the latter especially important for encouraging resilient feelings and behaviors. (For an excellent and highly entertaining perspective on successful aging, see also Vaillant, 2002.)

Conclusion

Much of the research reviewed in this chapter supports the proposition that older workers have the capacity to be successful on the job and, more broadly, to maintain job and life satisfaction well into older age. Positive correlations between age and job attitudes mean that older employees are likely to be more satisfied, committed, and involved in their jobs and, for the most part, easier to manage than younger employees because of their generally more tempered attitudes and more effective behaviors (e.g., citizenship).

In the area of personality, there are also reasons to be positive about potential contributions of older workers. Research suggests that on average older people are higher on traits desirable in work settings, such as conscientiousness and dependability, emotional stability, and agreeableness. The only negative finding in this regard is that older people are likely to be lower than younger people in openness to new experiences and behavioral flexibility.

Finally, we have seen that from a broader life satisfaction perspective, there are successful strategies for older adults to use. These include setting goals with flexibility built in, ensuring one's work and life environment are conducive to successful functioning, and maintaining social and interpersonal ties to make more likely resilient reactions to adversity.

5

Older Workers, Employment Patterns, and the Nature of Work

The workplace has been undergoing major changes over the past several decades. Globalization; organizational downsizing, "right-sizing," and restructuring; the use of information technology; changes in work contracts; and increased use of alternative work strategies and schedules have transformed the nature of work in many organizations. A growing number of older workers, female workers, and dual-career couples have also contributed to the change of the workforce. In this chapter we examine how the confluence of occupational trends, changing demographics, employment patterns, and job characteristics may shape the world of work over the next several decades.

Some researchers and workplace futurists have speculated that the world of work is in the midst of such fundamental change that there may be no stable jobs in the future. Work activities may be organized around projects and initiatives, with flexible task forces to deal with organizational requirements (e.g., Bridges, 1994). In such an environment, adequate job performance will require increased flexibility and adaptability in order to deal effectively with these less well-defined roles. Whether one embraces this perspective or not, the trend toward more flexible organizational structures and more adaptable organization members seems clear.

At the very least, these workforce changes are likely to result in different occupational and organizational structures in the future.

Technological modernization will require workers to adjust to new equipment and procedures, adapt to ever-changing environments, and continue to enhance their job-related skills. Technology changes the nature of work, and as Czaja (2001) has suggested, it will have a major impact on the future structure of the labor force, changing the jobs that are available and how they are performed.

If the occupational distribution of older workers in the labor force remains the same as it is currently, older workers will be employed in jobs and industries that are expected to continue expanding. However, this does not mean that such opportunities will necessarily be available for older workers. Factors such as job and skill requirements and negative stereotyping of older workers by employers and organizations influence such decisions. According to the Bureau of Labor Statistics' *Occupational Outlook Handbook* (U.S. Department of Labor, Bureau of Labor Statistics, 2003), almost two thirds of the projected job openings in the next 10 years will require some on-the-job training.

Changing technology is almost certain to change the structure of the labor force in the future. Czaja and Moen (2004) noted recently that in 2001 more than half of the labor force used a computer at work. This number is likely to increase as developments in technology continue. In fact, computer occupations such as software engineers, support specialists, and network and systems administrators will account for 8 out of the 20 fastest growing job areas, and the use of computers and other forms of technology is becoming more prevalent in other occupations as well (U.S. Department of Labor, Bureau of Labor Statistics, 2003). Not surprisingly, most workers, including older workers, will need to interact with some type of technology to perform their jobs.

It will also be important to understand how the spreading use of technology in most occupations will affect employment opportunities for older workers. Technology will create new jobs and opportunities for employment for some workers and eliminate jobs and create conditions of unemployment for others. It will also change the ways in which jobs are performed and alter job content and job demands. Workers will have to learn to use technical systems and new ways of performing jobs (Czaja & Moen, 2004).

Thus, workers will need to upgrade their knowledge, skills, and abilities to avoid problems with obsolescence, most likely learning new systems and new activities at multiple points during their working lives. Issues of skill obsolescence and worker retraining are highly significant for older workers, because they are less likely than younger workers to have had exposure to the latest technologies. According to Rosen and Jerdee (1985), some older workers may see technological change as a threat to their jobs and potentially an added burden from a retraining perspective; others are more upbeat about these changes and embrace the prospect of continuing education and training. Increased use of technology also tends to mean a reduction in the physical demands of work, a positive trend for the older worker, because any decline in muscular strength that might accompany aging would become less consequential.

Because organizations increasingly operate in wide and varied situations, cultures, and environments, not only will workers need to be more versatile and able to handle more diverse and complex tasks, but employers will need to deal with an increasingly diverse workplace. In the remainder of this chapter, we examine the role of the aging worker in terms of occupational trends and worker capabilities.

Employment Patterns of Older Workers

As we have noted, older workers are an ever-changing, heterogeneous pool of individuals. Changes in labor force composition as well as participation and retirement behavior have fundamentally altered the impact of key segments of this population over the past several decades and will continue to do so. Ongoing transformation to a more technology-driven and service-oriented economy and accompanying shifts in the occupational distribution of employment have altered the labor market within which the older worker must operate. These changes in the labor force and in the structure and function of jobs clearly influence the employment outlook for older workers (Sum & Fogg, 1990).

Occupational Trends

In chapter 1 we discussed the changing demographics of the workforce that point to a future shortage of younger employees and an increase in the number of older workers and in the proportion of women in the labor force. As older workers occupy a greater percentage of jobs in the coming years, these percentages will vary across different occupational groups. Because the Census Bureau and the Bureau of Labor Statistics routinely collect data on population and workforce trends, including occupational areas of growth and decline, it is relatively easy to project future employment patterns with some accuracy.

Hecker (2001) examined data collected for the calendar year 2000 across 10 primary occupational groups: management, business, and financial; professional and related occupations; services; sales and related occupations; office and administrative support; farming, fishing, and forestry; construction and extraction; installation, maintenance, and repair; production; and transportation and material moving occupations. He concluded that among these occupational groups, two in particular—professional occupations and services occupations—are expected to grow the fastest and add the most jobs between 2000 and 2010. Together, these two occupational groups should provide more than half of the total job growth in the economy for the first decade of the 21st century. On the other end of the continuum, the three slowest growing groups are expected to be office and administrative support occupations; production occupations; and farming, fishing, and forestry occupations.

As a result of the different growth rates among these 10 primary occupational groups, the total employment distribution should change to a certain extent by 2010, but the relative ranking of the groups by employment size is expected to stay the same (see Table 5.1). Professional and related occupations will continue to rank first; farming, fishing, and forestry occupations will continue to rank last. In fact, the projections suggest that only the professional and services occupational groups will improve their relative share of the labor market, adding almost 2.5 percentage points to its ranks during the 10-year period.

Table 5.1

Employment by Major Occupational Group, 2000 and 2010

		2000		2010		Change		Total job openings, 2000–2010[a]
Rank	Occupational group	N	%	N	%	N	%	
1	Professional	26,758	18.4	33,709	20.1	6,952	26.0	12,160
2	Services	26,075	17.9	31,162	18.6	5,008	19.5	13,505
3	Office and administrative support	23,882	16.4	26,053	15.5	2,171	9.1	7,667
4	Management, business, and finance	15,519	10.7	17,635	10.5	2,115	13.6	5,109
5	Sales	15,513	10.7	17,365	10.4	1,852	11.9	6,712
6	Production	13,060	9.0	13,811	8.2	750	5.7	3,932
7	Transportation and material moving	10,088	6.9	11,618	6.9	1,530	15.2	3,949
8	Construction and extraction	7,451	5.1	8,439	5.0	989	13.3	2,469
9	Installation, maintenance, and repair	5,820	4.0	6,482	3.9	662	11.4	1,944
10	Farming, fishing, and forestry	1,429	1.0	1,480	0.9	51	3.6	485

Note. Numbers are in thousands. Data extracted from the Bureau of Labor Statistics' Web site (www.bls.gov/emp).

[a]Includes openings related to growth and net replacement.

Within the professional and related occupations group, which are expected to add almost 7 million workers, nearly three fourths of the growth is projected to occur within three subgroups: computer and mathematical occupations; health care practitioners and technical occupations; and education, training, and library occupations. Computer and mathematical occupations (e.g., computer programmer, systems analyst, database administrator) are projected to add roughly 2 million employees and grow most rapidly among the eight professional and related occupations subgroups. This demand in computer-related occupations should continue for the foreseeable future. Health care practitioners and technical occupations are projected to add another 1.6 million jobs, because the demand for health care services continues to grow rapidly as well.

Between 2000 and 2010, employment in services occupations is expected to grow by over 5 million jobs. Of the subgroups making up the services occupations, food preparation and serving was the largest in 2000 and is also projected to add the most jobs by 2010. Health care support occupations (e.g., medical assistant, nursing aid) are expected to add over 1 million jobs; protective services (e.g., security guard, law enforcement worker) are also projected to grow rapidly.

In addition to growth trends in different occupations, the need for new workers also arises as replacements for those who leave their jobs to enter other occupations, retire, or leave the labor force for other reasons. According to Hecker (2001), in many occupations job openings that result from replacement exceed openings generated from employment growth. In fact, between 2000 and 2010, more job openings are expected to result from replacement needs (35.8 million) than from employment growth (22.2 million). Occupations like food preparation and serving, in part because of the limited training requirements and low pay, tend to generate relatively large numbers of job openings tied to replacement needs. Services occupations are projected to have the largest number of total job openings, roughly 13.5 million (see Table 5.1).

Occupational Trends and Older Workers

Older workers hold jobs in a wide range of occupations similar to those occupied by younger workers (see Table 5.2). Bovbjerg,

Jeszeck, and Petersen (2001), using a somewhat different occupational clustering strategy than Hecker (2001), provided a more detailed breakdown of employees by age and occupational group.[1] They found that relatively similar percentages of workers in all age groups (i.e., 30–39; 40–54, 55–64, and 65–74) were employed in white-collar occupations (i.e., executive, administrator, or manager; professional or technical; sales; administrative support). As can be seen in Table 5.2, these percentages ranged from 58.2 to 63.2, with the three older age categories less than 2 percentage points apart.

Bovbjerg et al. (2001) noted that the main differences in the employment distribution across the age groups can be found in services and blue-collar occupations. For example, although 14.5% of workers ages 65 to 74 are employed in service occupations, only 10.8% of workers ages 40 to 54 hold such jobs. In addition, 29.1% of workers ages 30 to 39 are employed in blue-collar occupations, whereas only 23.7% of workers ages 65 to 74 are similarly employed.

Table 5.3 provides a detailed look at the number of individuals within the two older age groups (55–64 and 65–74) that are employed in each of the major occupational groups. The table also provides information about the proportion of workers in each occupational group that comes from each of the two age groups. Workers ages 55 to 64 were a significant percentage of the total workforce—10.6% or slightly less than 14 million—in 2000. More individuals from the 55-to-64 age group can be found in professional and technical occupations than in any other occupational group and accounted for more than 2.6 million workers in 2000. It is also interesting to note that this age group contributed almost 19% of the workers to the professional and technical occupational group. The executive and manager occupations ranked second, with almost 2.4 million 55- to 64-year-old employees.

Workers ages 65 to 74 make up much smaller percentages of all 10 occupational groups. This is due, in part, to the fact that many in this age group have exited the labor force. As can be seen in Table 5.3, the four occupational groups most highly populated

---

[1]Hecker's (2001) occupational groupings reflect the 2000 Standard Occupational Classification system recently implemented. Bovbjerg et al.'s (2001) system grouping reflects the classification system used previously.

Table 5.2
Distribution of Occupational Groups Within Each Age Group

	Age group (years)			
Occupational group	30–39	40–54	55–64	65–74
Executive, administrator, manager	15.5	18.0	17.2	16.1
Professional and technical	19.6	20.8	19.0	15.4
Sales	10.6	10.7	11.6	15.5
Administrative support	12.8	13.7	13.9	15.4
White collar	58.5	63.2	61.7	62.4
Production, craft, repair	12.5	11.7	9.9	6.5
Farming, fishing, forestry	2.1	2.1	2.8	5.8
Transportation	4.6	4.0	4.7	5.6
Machine operator, assembly	6.2	5.6	5.0	3.1
Laborers, handlers	3.7	2.8	2.7	2.2
Blue collar	29.1	26.2	25.1	23.2
Services	12.5	10.8	13.2	14.5

Note. Data are percentages of an occupation within an age group. Data are derived from Bureau of Labor Statistics and Bureau of the Census data presented in Bovbjerg et al. (2001).

with 65- to 74-year-old employees are (a) executive, administrator, and manager; (b) sales; (c) professional and technical; and (d) administrative support. Each contributes just over half a million employees ages 65 or older. With the exception of farming, fishing, and forestry, where workers ages 65 to 74 constitute over 6% of that cluster, this age group accounts for less than 4% of the workers in any other occupational group.

Occupations and Older Workers' Abilities and Interests

Many older workers who reach retirement age do not completely withdraw from the labor force; instead, they switch from career jobs to other types of work. There may be several reasons for a

Table 5.3

Occupations of Workers Ages 55 Years and Older in 2000

Occupation	No. of workers		Workers in occupation (%)	
	55–64 years	65–74 years	55–64 years	65–74 years
Professional and technical	2,628,274	530,852	18.7	3.1
Executive, administrator, manager	2,376,268	553,003	12.0	2.8
Administrative support	1,927,958	529,227	10.5	2.9
Services	1,829,659	499,328	10.6	2.9
Sales	1,610,556	533,841	10.5	3.5
Production, craft, repair	1,367,729	223,508	9.4	1.5
Machine operator, assembly	695,672	105,748	9.3	1.4
Transportation	653,316	193,120	11.9	3.5
Farm, forestry, fishing	391,057	105,748	12.5	6.3
Laborers, handlers	374,737	74,724	7.2	1.4
All occupations	13,855,226	3,441,334	10.6	2.6

Note. Data are derived from Bureau of Labor Statistics and Bureau of the Census data presented in Bovbjerg et al. (2001).

shift in this occupational distribution as workers age. For example, workers in occupations with heavy physical requirements or stressful demands may not wish to continue in such jobs. Other workers may change jobs because they seek part-time work that is unavailable in their current occupation.

In the jobs held after such transfers, those who would like to continue working may not fully use their training, abilities, and interest, thus limiting their productive contribution (and their earnings). Muller and Knapp (2003) have suggested that such a potential mismatch between the requirements of the jobs and older workers' skills should be examined more closely. They believe this possible disparity is especially significant for society, given the increasing educational attainment and declining disability rates of aging cohorts in the United States.

To address this issue, Muller and Knapp (2003) identified jobs commonly held by older persons in the United States and examined worker abilities and worker interests characterized by those jobs. They first identified a set of 10 occupations where older workers (>65 years) are most commonly found. These 10 occupations are distributed across 7 of the 10 major occupational groups shown in Table 5.1. These jobs are composed of a wide variety of tasks, leading the authors to suggest that older workers are a heterogeneous group.

Then, using O*NET, a comprehensive Department of Labor database of worker and job attributes, Muller and Knapp (2003) analyzed two O*NET worker-specific descriptors—abilities and interests—and found six worker interests and 52 abilities. They included a broad range of physical and intellectual abilities, such as oral and written comprehension, reasoning, number facility, problem sensitivity, originality, fluency of ideas, memorization, manual dexterity, stamina, and dynamic strength.

They concluded that (a) numerous abilities are represented by the 10 occupations as a group; (b) the range of abilities within many of the occupations is great, that is, many of the occupations require a wide variety of abilities rather than just a few; and (c) worker interests, too, are diverse, with no single type of worker interest predominating as most representative of jobs where older workers are commonly found.

Muller and Knapp (2003) suggested that it is unclear whether the "important" jobs reflect preference by older workers or a lack of opportunity for other kinds of work. They noted that older workers' preference for workplace flexibility is a common theme in the literature relating to the employment of older persons. They suggested that older workers might be clustering around occupations that are characterized by some degree of flexibility, or perhaps the supply of such jobs is more limited than would be preferred by older workers. Each carries implications for how the labor force participation of older Americans could be made more consistent with both individual preferences and the financial side effects of life in an aging society.

Occupations and Retirement Patterns

In chapter 1, we discussed reasons for staying in or leaving the workforce. Retirement patterns also tend to vary by industry. For example, workers in manufacturing are more likely to be unionized and have greater access to pension benefits, which contributes to retirement decisions. In addition, the more physically demanding jobs tend to lead to earlier retirements than do occupations that require less physical labor. Workers with physically demanding occupations are more likely to be found in some industries than others. For example, almost two thirds of workers in manufacturing are craftsmen or operators and laborers. In contrast, business and personal services; public administration; and finance, insurance, and real estate industries are less likely to employ persons in these occupations (Uccello, 1998).

Dohm (2000) suggested that replacement needs between 2003 and 2008 will be almost 25% larger than they were between 1993 and 1998, underscoring the potential significance of retirement by the baby boom cohort. By 2008, the oldest baby boomers will be age 62; thus, the period between 2003 and 2008 will include baby boomers ages 45 to 62. Dohm examined the occupations and industries likely to be most affected when the oldest baby boomers begin to retire. Among the broad occupation groups, the executive, administrative, and managerial occupations are expected to experience the greatest turnover. Workers age 45 and older make up 41% of the workers in this group, and 42% of these older workers are expected to leave the workforce by 2008. That amounts to nearly 3 million job openings in this occupational group alone and could result in a significant loss of managerial skills and experience.

Occupations within the professional and technical group will also be seriously affected, and the industry within this occupational group that will be most affected by baby boomer retirements is educational services. Nearly all the major occupations that make up this industry have people who retire at a relatively young age (because of pensions that often provide full coverage for qualified employees after 30 years of service). In addition, hiring cutbacks during the 1980s and 1990s raised the average age of workers in the teaching professions, leaving relatively fewer workers to move into the expected vacancies.

Transportation occupations (e.g., railroads, bus service, urban transit, taxicab service, air transportation) will also be hit hard. The health care services and construction industry are two other sectors that have at least eight occupations that will experience heavy baby boomer retirement. Dohm (2000) also suggested that the effect of baby boomer retirements will be more dramatic in the decade following 2008. By 2018, all but the youngest baby boomers will be of retirement age.

So even if the trend toward early retirement has indeed reversed, as some have suggested, particular industries will still feel the impact of the aging population on their labor pools, because older workers are not evenly distributed across all industries. These sectors with a "retirement bulge," or a large portion of their current workforce that will reach the customary retirement age during the next decade, and those industries that face a "youth squeeze" because they depend heavily on a contracting supply of young workers, will likely come under increased labor market pressures to expand their employment of older workers.

The organizations with a retirement bulge may be encouraged to adopt more flexible retirement practices and to restructure some jobs so that their experienced workers can be retained rather than retired. Similarly, firms experiencing a youth squeeze as the size of the pool of young labor entrants begins to shrink may seek older workers as a source of replacement labor (Doeringer & Terkla, 1990).

Final Thoughts About Occupational Trends and Older Workers

Using Bureau of Labor Statistics and Census data, Bovbjerg et al. (2001) projected that between 2000 and 2008, the number and percentage of workers age 55 and older should increase across all major occupational categories because of the aging of the workforce. The largest change for this age group is expected to occur in white-collar occupations (see Figure 5.1). For example, the percentage of the workers age 55 and over in professional and technical occupations will grow substantially, from 22% to 29%. Among executive and manager occupations, the percentage of workers age 55 and older is also projected to rise steadily, from 15% to 23%. The smallest change should occur in services occupations, as the percentage of the workforce age 55 and older that is employed in the services sector remains relatively stable. The change in the percentage of workers in each major occupational category identified by Bovbjerg et al. who are age 55 and older is shown in Figure 5.1.

Some general statements can be made about aging workers and their occupations. As workers age, their occupational migration tends to be toward white-collar and services occupations and away from physically demanding occupations. This shift from blue-collar to white-collar occupations is expected to continue for the foreseeable future. Several factors might contribute to this shift. First, as workers age they may experience health problems that diminish their ability to perform their jobs; therefore, some choose to move to less physically demanding jobs. Second, those employees who choose to stay in the workplace to older ages tend to have held white-collar jobs throughout their careers.

The shift toward white-collar occupations can also be attributed to educational levels among the baby-boom cohort. As noted by Korczyk (2002), baby boomers are the most college-educated generation currently in the workforce. They are more likely to have completed some college or attained associate degrees, other vocational degrees, or bachelor's degrees than any other group between the ages of 25 and 65. Presently, 57% of persons between the ages of 40 and 54 have at least some college education compared with 42% of individuals ages 55 to 74. The greater level of educational attainment among the baby boomers may also mean that they have a broader range of jobs available to them than the current generation of older workers (Bovbjerg et al., 2001). Indeed, as Hecker (2001) reported, of the 30 fastest growing occupations, 21 require a postsecondary degree.

Job Characteristics and the Older Worker

In the first part of this chapter, we discussed general occupational trends and how the changing workplace might affect older workers' employment possibilities and occupational choices. In the

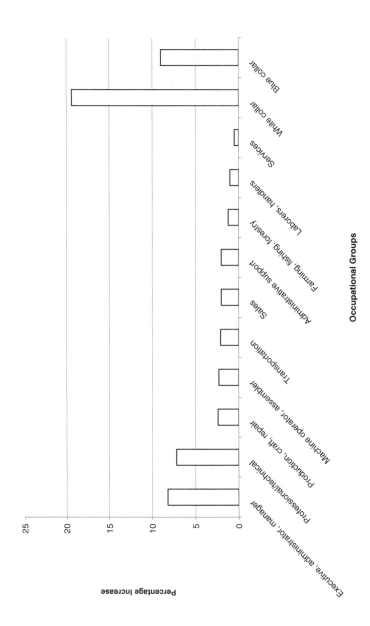

Figure 5.1. Increase in percentage of workers age 55 and older in major occupations between 2000 and 2008. Data are derived from Bovbjerg et al. (2001).

sections that follow we discuss how the characteristics and requirements of jobs may interact with the aptitudes and experiences of older workers either to facilitate or to hinder job performance. Certainly, jobs and tasks can be categorized in a variety of ways that may have different implications for older workers. However, within the context of broad categorizations of jobs and workers, it is important to remember our discussion of age stereotyping in chapter 2 and guard against overgeneralization.

Recall that we discussed the notion that some jobs or tasks may be perceived as more suited for certain age groups, and employees whose chronological age does not match the stereotypical age may be adversely affected in terms of job rewards. The reminder here, before we look more closely at what the research has to say about matching older worker capabilities and interests with job requirements, is that one cannot forget that perceptions can play a major role in categorizing older workers and consequently the employment opportunities available to them.

Job Complexity and Cognitive Demands

Warr (1994) proposed a classification system based on job experience and age-based skill decay to clarify relationships between age and performance in different types of jobs. He suggested that occupations vary in the extent to which (a) job experience results in higher levels of job performance and (b) specific skills required for successful performance declines with age. The combination of these two variables produces four possible outcomes.

The first category, which Warr (1994) labeled *Type A activities*, involves tasks and activities with cognitive demand requirements that can be met by the employee despite advancing age. In addition, the performance of Type A activities is enhanced through experience. The acquisition of interpersonal skills and social knowledge as a result of accumulated experience falls into this group. This category, then, represents activities with positive associations between age and job performance, because the situations are relatively stable, and knowledge and skills can continue to be developed by older workers.

A second category, labeled *Type B activities*, includes situations where work activities are relatively routine and nonproblematic.

These activities demand either a limited skill set or skills that are firmly established so that behavior is fairly automatic. In such circumstances, differences in task performance are not expected across age groups.

Type C activities are those that older people may have increasing difficulties with because of some decline in information processing skills or physical capacities. Nonetheless, overall performance is not degraded because workers find ways to compensate for any physical or cognitive decrement through acquired experience. These types of activities are very common in jobs.

The last grouping, *Type D activities*, includes tasks characterized by continuous rapid information processing or some kind of demanding physical activity that become more difficult with advancing age. In these situations, some of the basic capacities available to the older worker may be exceeded, and situational experiences are of little help. Activities in this group are often found in jobs whose content changes rapidly, so that previous knowledge and skills may easily become obsolete. Type D activities encompass a relatively small portion of job behaviors.

Warr's (1994) classification scheme is one useful way to categorize tasks and activities based on the potential impact of the aging process. A useful next step would be a grouping of occupations based on the four-category system and the tasks and activities the occupations are characterized by. Warr suggested that older workers are at a disadvantage only in jobs or occupations that require Type D activities.

Influence of Jobs on Aging

Although Warr's (1994) categorization scheme examines the ways in which age-related processes can affect behaviors at work, looking at the aging process–work performance causal linkage in the reverse direction can also be useful. Baltes and Baltes (1990a) have suggested that some environments may be more conducive to successful aging than others. There is evidence that complex environmental conditions that foster learning and require the application of problem-solving skills can have a positive effect on the intellectual functioning of older individuals still in the workforce (Schooler, Caplan, & Oates, 1998). The idea is that complex environments expose the worker to a wider array of stimuli and greater ambiguity than do simple environments. In addition, they often require the individual to consider more options when making decisions. By presenting more challenges and requiring more complicated information-processing activity, complex environments embody the types of experience and training that foster superior cognitive functioning.

Kohn and Schooler (1983) began a longitudinal study in the early 1960s on the psychological effects of occupational conditions. They found that job conditions that offer a challenge and the opportunity to do self-directed, complex work tend to increase intellectual flexibility. Conversely, work conditions that limit intellectual challenge and self-direction on the job tend to decrease intellectual flexibility. Schooler, Mulatu, and Oates (1999) followed up the Kohn and Schooler work and replicated these findings with the same participants 20 years after the original study was conducted. Not only did they confirm the assumption that the degree to which substantively complex work increases intellectual flexibility remains constant over the life span, but they also discovered that the complexity of the work people do tends to increase with age.

The argument here is that more complex jobs provide employees with challenge and stimulation that can lead to the enhancement of skill development over time, whereas jobs with low levels of complexity that involve simple, highly routine activities may lead to a deterioration in work performance over time. Thus, workers in more challenging jobs that require the continuous use and practice of critical cognitive abilities are more able to perform effectively into older age (Farr, Tesluk, & Klein, 1998).

Additional support for such an argument comes from a meta-analysis by Waldman and Avolio (1986). They found that the type of work performed appears to moderate the relationship between age and performance, with a stronger negative relationship between age and work performance being found for those in nonprofessional jobs as compared to those in professional jobs. It should be noted, however, that McEvoy and Cascio (1989) did not replicate this finding in a subsequent meta-analysis. Later, Avolio, Waldman, & McDaniel (1990) found that performance tended to level off or decline more quickly for employees in low-level clerical jobs than it did in higher craft and service types of occupations. Sparrow and Davies (1988) found that for all age groups in the study, performance was higher for the more complex tasks. In addition, job performance peaked on complex tasks at a significantly higher average age. Certainly, as noted by McEvoy and Cascio, because of the relatively small number of studies available that contain workers over 60 years of age, much additional research is needed on the 50- to 70-year-old age cohort.

Still, as reflected in Warr's four-category framework, there may be limits on how much job complexity can help maintain effective performance as workers age. He suggested that there may be a range of optimal levels of cognitive complexity and cognitive demands beyond which performance does not improve, or may even decline, especially when extremely high levels of processing and working memory demands in terms of decision-making speed, concentration, and problem solving are involved.

Conclusion

In a recent study examining factors influencing retirement, Uccello (1998) found that the ability of workers to extend their working lives depends on the nature of their jobs. Workers with more physically demanding jobs retire earlier than those with less physically demanding jobs. Similarly, Hayward, Grady, Hardy, and Sommers (1989) found that workers in jobs that are cognitively demanding and less physically demanding are less likely to retire than those in jobs with low substantive complexity and high physical demands. They also found that health limitations have a strong impact on the decision to retire (Czaja, 2001).

With increasing age, many workers migrate toward jobs that have more desirable characteristics, as a result of which they might be expected to be more satisfied. Older workers may also gain greater discretion over their work activities and thus become better able to control activities and events. Satisfaction and control may arise from promotion to more senior jobs or from increased tenure in a single job or may be associated with norms about the treatment of older workers. Warr (1998) suggested that the opportunity to use valued abilities has also been shown to be crucial to the job-related mental health of workers. However, through gradual obsolescence and more limited learning and relearning opportunities as workers age, some older employees may have only limited chances to use high skill levels. Older workers also tend to seek more variety from their jobs as well. Unfortunately, as their activities and skills become increasingly specialized, on average, this feature is often reduced for older workers. In response to these individual and organizational forces that influence work and retirement decisions of older workers, H. L. Sterns and Gray (1999) advocated greater career self-management, a topic we discuss in detail in the chapters that follow.

The world of work is undergoing major change, not the least of which is the aging of the workforce. Changing retirement patterns; changing occupational trends, fueled by ever-evolving technological innovations; and changing motivations and capabilities of workers as they age, mean the human resources landscape of tomorrow will be vastly different and more challenging than it is today. All of these changes point to a need to develop strategies that better allow for successful integration of older workers into the workforce. To optimize utilization of the older worker, organizational human resources specialists need to gain a better understanding of issues surrounding older workers, including skills and knowledge obsolescence, the need for development of new knowledge and skills, the importance of creating new opportunities for employment, and the need to find ways to motivate and reward different age groups in the workforce.

6

Older Workers and Human Resource Management Policies and Practices

The aging workforce presents organizations with numerous challenges that will become more pronounced over the next several decades. As the baby boomers swell the ranks of those on the cusp of retirement, the average age of the working population will increase substantially. Definitions of what constitutes *old* or *older* have shifted over the years as a result of increasing life expectancy and more active and productive lifestyles. With the mass entry of the baby boom cohort into the 45-to-64 age group, these workers will become central to the economy as a whole, and more specifically to human resource (HR) planning. As a large number of the baby boomers reach "normal" retirement age, many of them indicate that they may delay retirement or work well into it. Consequently, people past traditional retirement age will make up an ever larger part of the labor pool. In this chapter we introduce the notion that organizations must begin to invest in HR strategies that actively address the needs and desires of older segments of the workforce.

In previous chapters, we have discussed forces that contribute to early retirement and forces that encourage delayed retirement. We have also talked about how the nature of work is changing in ways that affect older workers in particular and discussed age discrimination that confronts an aging workforce. These challenges will affect employer policies and practices, especially as they relate to hiring, training, retaining, promoting, assigning jobs to, and terminating older workers. If organizations are to adapt successfully to these changing workforce dynamics, they must ensure that their organizational policies and actions are designed in ways that encourage and promote continued investment in older employees.

The looming retirement of the baby boomers is projected to have a large impact on all sectors of the economy. The question then becomes, "What is being done to ensure continuity of leadership, knowledge, and expertise so that productivity and (maybe even) organizational survival is not jeopardized in the future?"

Strategic HR planning is essential to ensure that the people and competencies are in place to meet these needs. It is essential that organizations begin planning now to address labor shortages. Workforce planning should include such things as analyzing the demographics of the workforce, reviewing turnover statistics and retirement projections, and developing strategies to meet current and future needs. Innovation and flexibility in responding to the labor force challenge of the 21st century will be a key source of competitive advantage for organizations.

Organizational Policies and Procedures

In recent years, federal legislation has been enacted that allows employees to work beyond traditional retirement ages. Anticipating a significant decline in the ratio of workers to retirees when the baby boomers retire, Social Security regulations have been rewritten to encourage delay of labor force withdrawal and to reduce financial incentives for early retirement. In addition, age discrimination laws have been extended to protect workers from mandatory retirement at any age. Nonetheless, many organizations continue to be enamored with downsizing and restructuring activities, moves that often affect older workers disproportionately (Shea, 1991). Corporate policies that for decades encouraged workforce turnover to permit early retirement of older people and recruitment of younger talent have been good for employers (and sometimes good for employees as well). However, they run counter to the policies and practices that are needed to cope with future shortages of talent and experience (Robson, 2001).

Until relatively recently, few organizations have concentrated on developing and implementing unique policies and practices involving older workers. That is because retirement targets used to be relatively standardized. The traditional employer viewpoint concerning career progression patterns has been that employees would remain relatively productive until they reach retirement at age 65 or earlier. In instances where management had concerns about the possibility of older employee productivity decline, management understood that patience would be rewarded in that such employees will retire in the not-too-distant future. Now, however, most employees can continue to work until at least age 70 if they so desire, and a significant minority of older workers appear to want to continue working in some capacity.

As we move rapidly toward the baby boomer retirement years, a strategic HR management challenge will be to create new and attractive opportunities that capture the desire of older workers to make significant organizational contributions. These opportunities may involve part-time work, job redesign, organizational retraining, and alternative career paths. To meet these challenges, organizations need to create structures, policies, and procedures that foster an environment supportive of older workers' performance, work attitudes and motivation, and physical and psychological well-being. Unfortunately, most organizations are ill-prepared to meet the challenges associated with older workers.

Friedan (1993), for example, described a survey conducted by the American Society for Personnel Administration in 1988. Responses were gathered from representatives of more than 600 organizations concerning problems with managing an older workforce and whether their companies had adopted policies to address these current and future problems. Forty-seven percent of respondents reported "moderate to serious problems" with managing the careers of senior employees. Less than 10% of these administrators believed that their own companies had policies to accommodate the needs of older employees who wanted to stay on the job in either a full-time or part-time capacity.

More recently, in a survey conducted by the AARP (AARP Work Link Team Program, 2000), 400 senior managers were asked to rate important employment issues; they rated "the aging of the workforce" issue at 4.5 out of 10, which was 6th on a list of 10 issues. In other words, it appears that HR managers are not yet particularly concerned about this issue. In addition, few of those surveyed were able to identify steps their companies were taking to address the issue.

As organization managers begin to realize that they must address the needs of older workers with appropriate HR strategies, they should closely examine their current personnel selection, retention, and promotion procedures and soundly ground them in science and law. Managers must be especially careful to avoid using age considerations when recruiting and selecting employees, offering training and development opportunities to workers, and promoting employees. Decisions regarding employee transfers, demotions, and terminations must also be based on performance or potential, not employee age. Managers must examine company policies and management practices for potential legal problems and identify and resolve situations in which age discrimination may play a role before complaints are filed and litigation occurs (Dennis, 1988b).

HR professionals must also understand that, whereas management systems can offer older workers opportunity for challenging job responsibilities and motivate them to pursue learning and self-development activities, these systems are influenced by an organization's norms and stereotypes toward older workers (Farr, Tesluk, & Klein, 1998). In turn, an organization's culture affects its policies and practices. As we have discussed earlier in this book, age-related stereotypes abound within organizations, and if these norms and stereotypes are a part of the general culture of the organization, they may influence decisions regarding pay, promotions, assignments, and training opportunities.

Although the corporate culture regarding older workers cannot be changed overnight, over time an organization's HR policies and practices can begin to alter culture, aging stereotypes, norms, and values. Because managers influence the development or change of an organization's cultural values, they can play a critical role in moving the organization to an age-neutral environment, one that is supportive of age-friendly policies and practices. For example, Farr et al. (1998) suggested that requiring managers to attend age-related training may serve to decrease age-stereotyping and discrimination. Moreover, if training programs are provided for all employees and are not limited to certain age groups, a culture is created that values learning and employee growth.

Generally, then, it is incumbent on employers and managers to increase their own knowledge, skills, and attitudes that contribute to effective HR management of a diverse, maturing workforce. Certainly, this requires a greater understanding of the links between employee motivation, organizational incentives, and productivity. Management plays a key role in promoting awareness of how company policies and practices enable a diverse workforce to perform most effectively. The development and implementation of effective HR management practices for the aging workforce are critical, and organizations that have developed flexible and positive policies and practices for the management of older employees should have a decided marketplace advantage.

Organizations also need to have a better understanding of the organization's workforce profile, including its current age structure, and how that might impact various organizational policies and practices. For example, an organization might make very different decisions about its career development practices and succession planning activities for a relatively old workforce compared with a relatively young workforce. Recently, a survey of 150 senior HR executives found that 66% of the participants reported that their companies had no age profile of their workforce, resulting in a complete lack of hard data about how retirements will affect their businesses (Munson, 2003). At a time when new HR management software is available for producing and monitoring the demographic profile of a workforce, such data would seem relatively easy for organizations to collect.

Human Resource Management Strategies and the Older Worker

The late-career years present numerous opportunities and challenges for individuals and organizations. Although the literature suggests that aging tends to result in some physiological declines during the later stages of careers, these declines do not necessarily affect job performance, as has been discussed in chapter 3.

Certainly, older workers tend to have accumulated a wealth of skills, experience, and organizational savvy that can be quite useful. For example, Beehr and Bowling (2002) noted that older workers may make excellent mentors for newer employees or serve as valuable advisors and sounding boards for decision makers in the organization.

Thus, when employees are in the later stages of their careers, organizations should take advantage of their numerous capabilities. Employers should recognize that most employees who plan to work in retirement hope to build on their accumulated expertise by remaining in a line of work that is similar to their current occupation. Employers should actively tap into this labor pool's talent and expertise while keeping in mind that new experiences are valued by many older workers. Unless organizations find ways to retain aging boomers' skills and experience, productivity in organizations is bound to suffer. If older workers choose to leave the organization, their skills, abilities, and experiences may serve them well as consultants and may be quite useful to their former employers, or to the larger industry within which they worked.

Although Beehr and Bowling (2002) focused on the positive aspects of aging employees' "accumulated wisdom," it is also important to note the downside of losing this "institutional knowledge" as workers retire. Schetagne (2001) has suggested that only a small part of knowledge and skills is transmitted from older to younger workers before they leave the organization. This is especially true when early retirement options are used; workers are often given only a few weeks to a few months to decide whether to accept. As a result, it is difficult to imagine that such workers had time to transfer their on-the-job knowledge and experience to their younger colleagues. Of special concern should be the burgeoning retirement of baby boomers over the next few years, which may exacerbate this loss of institutional knowledge.

Schetagne (2001) argued that of all the available HR strategies and practices, the most important should be those that favor the transfer of knowledge and skills between generations of workers. Whether they take the form of financial support for training or a mentoring program between an older worker on the verge of retirement and a younger worker, these strategies, policies, and practices should encourage the transfer of knowledge and acquired skills from older workers to their younger successors.

It seems clear that different approaches and different policies of work are necessary to take full advantage of the talents of these workers moving into later career stages. A number of authors have suggested that many workers nearing age 50 may prefer increased flexibility of schedule and varied work opportunities. Thus, late career considerations may include such options as job sharing, phased retirement, and training and mentoring opportunities.

The availability of creative career management practices may be particularly important to members of the baby boom generation who are now beginning to be classified as older workers. Farr et al. (1998) have suggested that these workers, as they move into the latter stages of their careers, appear to be less focused on hierarchical advancement in the organization. Rather, they seem more oriented toward making use of their potential, developing new skill sets, and being challenged in their job assignments and responsibilities. As Morris and Venkatesh (2000) have suggested, management strategies that treat the "workforce" as a monolithic entity, with no real appreciation of differences across age groups, are likely to fail.

Selection, Placement, and Alternative Work Arrangements

A variety of HR management strategies have been suggested that offer older workers opportunities for flexible work scheduling, developing new knowledge and skills, or using their current skills and abilities set differently. They may include such personnel activities as job rotation or lateral job options, where employees are allowed to move to different jobs with similar levels of responsibility. Some organizations have strategies where older employees are given special assignments that require a high level of organization-specific knowledge, the type that older employees have gathered over the years. These job placement practices can be an extremely functional way of using older workers, because older employees can be given assignments that match their particular interests and talents.

Other creative HR management strategies may also be used, such as offering older workers certain choices of work arrangements, as they approach retirement age. These options would represent alternatives to the jobs they have been in over a period of years. A choice in work arrangements for older workers may permit those experiencing health problems or skill obsolescence to work more productively (Barth, McNaught, & Rizzi, 1995).

Two innovative, part-time forms of employment include job-sharing and phased retirement programs. *Job sharing* usually involves the sharing of one full-time job by two part-time workers, neither of whom is interested in working full-time. Job sharing, when it involves an older worker and a younger worker, might also facilitate the "transfer of knowledge" that we mentioned earlier. *Phased retirement* is typically used as an employment option for full-time employees who are several years away from retirement. These employees are permitted to reduce their work hours gradually, through shorter workdays or fewer days per year, to some minimum schedule until retirement. The concept underlying the use of phased retirement is that workers can "phase" into retirement gradually rather than work full-time until the day they retire (Paul, 1988).

Training

Training is another important element of strategic HR policies for older workers. Skill obsolescence may be particularly problematic for workers, especially in certain technology-intensive occupations. In fact, as noted by Farr et al. (1998), the pace of change of the work environment may set off a negative spiral for older workers related to their self-efficacy around developing new knowledge and skills, keeping pace with new work practices as they are implemented, developing new knowledge and skills, and subsequent job performance. Keeping skills fresh through training throughout the career life cycle is critical, but some studies have suggested that older workers may be less likely to participate in training programs than younger workers, either because they may be more hesitant, or because employers may not encourage them to participate.

H. L. Sterns and Doverspike (1988) suggested that employers may also be reluctant to hire persons over age 40 and offer them training. Thus, even though the large majority of older workers are healthy, dependable, and productive and have low accident rates, this reluctance to invest in older workers remains. Older workers sometimes contribute to this situation by their reluctance to volunteer for training or retraining because they feel uncertain about their ability to succeed in a training program or fear competition with younger workers. Now, and in the future, HR professionals must extend training opportunities to older workers and encourage them to participate.

Pay and Benefits

In addition to manipulating job responsibilities and assignments or offering training opportunities, sometimes a rethinking of existing pay and benefits can make a big difference to older workers. For example, Robson (2001) noted that large profit-sharing bonuses or options may have unintended effects, allowing employees to "buy more leisure" by retiring early or shifting to jobs with shorter hours. Some pension plans may provide early retirees with more in lifetime benefits, essentially encouraging their departure. Other plans may result in no additional benefits after a certain stage, in which case the drop in effective compensation may again encourage workers into retirement. For example, life insurance benefits may be less attractive to older workers who no longer have young dependents. Consequently, these employers can use knowledge of such preferences to think more innovatively about what forms of compensation are appealing to older workers.

Extended health benefits are one possibility. Some older employees may be particularly attracted to improved health insurance or other medical benefits. In fact, they may want to work beyond normal retirement age in order to keep their health insurance coverage. Although older people are healthier than they used to be, certain chronic conditions become more common with age. Consequently, HR professionals who seek older workers to fill part-time and consulting positions (which often do not come with health care benefits) may want to consider adding health care as a major incentive (Wellner, 2002).

Investing in the Older Worker

An organization's personnel practices often are driven by its HR philosophy. This philosophy may view older workers as "goods" with a limited usefulness, or it may view workers as "assets" that continue to grow if managed properly. In the face of increasing needs for technical, administrative, executive, and professional people, as well as service workers in most fields, and with projected shortages of younger people over the next 25 years, organizations should begin to focus more attention on developing and implementing strategies to foster continued use of older employees (Friedan, 1993).

All too often organizations yield to the temptation to "retire" older workers and replace them with younger, cheaper labor. Wages and salaries, for example, tend to increase up until age 50 or so and then level off, meaning that older workers are more costly than younger workers from a straight compensation perspective. During mergers and periods of corporate downsizing, the potential dollars saved by reducing the numbers of highly paid older workers have considerable appeal, although the appeal often has a short-term focus.

Surprisingly, however, companies rarely attempt to systematically analyze the costs and benefits of supporting employees in the latter stages of their careers (Rosen & Jerdee, 1985). Those who argue in favor of divesting their workforce of older employees tend to overlook the costs of recruiting and training new workers. These costs may be minimal if unskilled workers are available and needed, but they can be substantial when highly experienced workers are sought. Employers may also incur additional costs associated with relocating new workers, assisting spouses in finding work, and reduced productivity associated with the time required of workers to adjust to their new work environment. Rix (1990) reinforced the notion of such cost–benefit analysis by suggesting that the costs of retraining (rather than retiring) older workers should be balanced against replacement costs, which include recruitment, relocation, and training of new workers.

Simpson, Greller, and Stroh (2002) examined this notion that human capital investment is not and should not be made for people in late career. Although they noted that late career has been relatively understudied, they suggested that until recently, the only consensus that had emerged across the social science and public policy literature has been that employers were reluctant to train older workers, and in fact tended to offer them less on-the-job training than their younger co-workers. The following explanations have been offered for this phenomenon: (a) *opportunity costs* (experienced older workers are too valuable in their current jobs to allow the lost productivity resulting from time devoted to training); (b) *wage rates* (older workers are usually at the high end of the wage scale, so allowing them to spend time on training instead of their job incurs higher cost in wages than it does for younger persons); and (c) *expected payback period* (older employees have fewer remaining years of employment with the firm compared with younger employees). These combined effects lead employers to avoid making additional investments in their older workers.

Simpson et al. (2002) suggested that the notion of payback period is both arbitrary and unrealistic, noting that few human capital investments are expected to produce returns over the entire remainder of a person's career. More realistically, if the payback period is the 3 to 5 years that HR management professionals typically use to evaluate training investments, then a 55-year-old and a 25-year-old both can expect to be employed for the full period. They also suggested that the idea that the training of older workers is too expensive in terms of opportunity cost and wages is applicable only to on-the-job training. A more comprehensive perspective that includes all work-related educational activity (on the job, at the job, or off the job) does not support this proposition.

Yeatts, Folts, and Knapp (2000) recently discussed two philosophical models that represent HR management practices. They labeled these two approaches the *depreciation model* and the *conservation model*. The depreciation model implies that an individual's value to an organization peaks early in a career, levels off at midcareer, and steadily declines until retirement. In this

model, investment in older workers is viewed as cost-prohibi-
tive. Consequently, older employees in organizations with this
philosophy would be expected to receive little help in adapting
to workplace changes; they might even be offered incentives to
leave the organization. The alternative approach is the conservation model, which views employees of all ages as renewable assets that yield a high rate of return over long periods of time if
they are adequately educated, trained, and managed. In contrast
to the depreciation model, the conservation model can be expected
to result in older worker–friendly personnel practices that assist
employees in maintaining an acceptable fit with their jobs.

It makes considerable sense for organizations to adopt HR strategies that actively address the needs and desires of older segments of the workforce. Surveys have shown that, from the older
workers' perspective, there is a desire to continue working and
to have viable work options later in life. For example, a recent
survey by the AARP (Montenegro, Fisher, & Remez, 2002) found
that 84% of respondents (45–74 years of age) said they would work
even if they were financially set for life, and 69% said they planned
to work into their "retirement years." However, these older workers expressed a desire to work in ways different than what may
have defined their earlier careers. They wanted more flexibility
and autonomy in their work. They also suggested that their motivations for working are wide ranging—not only for the money
and health care coverage but also peace of mind, enjoyment, and
a sense of purpose.

When survey respondents were asked about how they would
like to finish out the latter stages of their careers, more than a
quarter said that during retirement they planned to work because
they enjoy working. Similarly, 24% said that they would work
because it was something interesting to do. In addition, 22% said
they would work for financial reasons, whereas 20% and 16%,
respectively, cited a desire to stay physically and mentally active.
These responses reflect a relatively new but increasingly common orientation among late-stage workers for "bridge jobs" or
flexible career jobs that offer new experiences or provide work–
life flexibility between careers or prior to retiring.

Additional insight into the motivations of these older workers
can be found in their responses to what they would want in an

ideal job. Respondents listed a chance to use their skills and talents (94%) and an opportunity to do something new (88%) as two job attributes they would desire in an ideal job. They also noted that such a job should allow "adequate" paid time off (86%); a flexible schedule (76%); health care benefits (84%); and good pension benefits (76%).

Respondents noted their concerns about current age discrimination. Sixty-seven percent of all respondents said they believed that age discrimination exists in the workplace, revealing a concern about opportunities to reenter the workplace and advance in their current jobs as they aged. A large percentage (60%) also said that they believed that older workers are the first to go when employers make cuts (Montenegro et al., 2002).

Another more recent study by AARP (2003) found that although many pre-retirees still talk about spending more time with loved ones, receiving pension and social security benefits, and engaging in activities they previously had no time for, a new, more multifaceted vision of retirement is emerging. Specifically, when asked to describe their personal definition of retirement, more than 70% of older workers yet to retire included "some form of work" as part of their personal definition of retirement.

Moreover, when asked to indicate why they have decided to work in their retirement years, pre-retirees and working retirees identified nonfinancial reasons such as staying mentally and physically active and remaining productive or useful. However, when respondents were forced to select a single factor in their decision to work, the need for money is mentioned as the primary motivator.

Conclusion

As the world of work becomes more influenced by technology and global concerns, change—and the pace of change—accelerates. This has given rise to the concept of learning as a career-long process. Some authors have urged a move away from the notion of training and retraining and toward the concept of continual learning. The organization that adopts this learning and performance perspective for all its employees will have created an HR management philosophy and practice where older workers will be among those striving for skill updating and performance improvement.

From a long-term perspective, HR practices can play a critical role in determining the types of experiences individuals accumulate over the course of their career. By exposing employees to a variety of situations and responsibilities, continual learning of critical knowledge and skills help ensure continued motivation to learn, positive work attitudes, and effective job performar;ce (Farr et al., 1998).

Although labor force participation rates drop sharply during the early 60s, particularly at ages 62 and 65, a substantial minority do work beyond 65. There is some evidence suggesting that the trend toward earlier retirement has leveled off, but most analysts agree that it is still likely that a significant number of people will opt for early retirement in the decades ahead. Compared with what is known about determinants of labor force participation among those in their early to mid-60s, relatively little is known about those who elect to work well beyond this age.

For policy makers and HR strategists looking for ways to increase labor force participation rates among those who are beyond retirement age, much remains to be learned about why at least some workers currently remain at work through their late 60s and into their 70s, and others choose to leave. A greater understanding of why different groups work beyond the typical age of retirement would help to provide a basis for developing policies targeted toward each group (Williamson & McNamara, 2001). Certainly, no one standard policy can hope to encourage labor force participation equally for all groups.

Because both private and public pensions helped to lower the average age of retirement in the past, it is reasonable to believe that modifications to existing practices can help to raise it again in the future. The goal will be to encourage more employees to remain in the workforce until retirement age and beyond, whether on a full-time basis or some other arrangement. Public policies and private practices that support continued involvement in productive work by older workers will go far toward meeting the challenges that lie ahead (see, e.g., Bass, Quinn, & Burkhauser, 1995).

It seems clear that in designing and implementing HR management policies, the needs and preferences of older workers must be considered. Career paths and career ladders should be designed to suit the needs of specific age groups. In the chapters that follow, we talk in greater detail about programs and strategies for reinvesting in older workers.

7

Organizational Strategies for Attracting, Utilizing, and Retaining Older Workers

Organizations are largely unprepared for the challenges that an aging workforce will bring. In preceding chapters we detailed the demographic forces at work, the social and organizational implications of those forces, and the population that will soon take center stage in the workforce—aging baby boomers. In this chapter and the next, we offer some solutions for organizations that wish to prepare for this new world of work.

Meeting these impending challenges is not simply an issue for employers. Such sweeping change will envelop not only employers, but government (e.g., in relation to policies); unions; and, of course, workers themselves. This chapter and the next offer a broad base of solutions that touch all parties in the employment relationship. It must be said at the outset, however, that solutions to many issues surrounding the aging workforce are not yet clear. Society, business, and science have been slow to react, but the urgency of the situation will soon be felt, as a predominant "culture of aging" quickly comes to the fore from the same group that so impacted the United States with the "culture of youth" in the 1960s and 1970s (Novelli, 2002).

In this chapter we first discuss some basic organizational requirements that must be in place for an organization to fully utilize the talents of older workers and be sensitive to their needs. These include a strong commitment from top management, efforts to actively combat age-based stereotypes and age norms, managerial training, and organizational support resources for older workers. In addition, we describe flexible work arrangements and compensation plans geared to the needs of older workers and the targeted recruitment of older workers. We then turn to issues pertaining to job placement of older workers, including selection and job design.

Organizational Requirements

Liebig (1988) summarized the organizational context necessary for effective utilization of the aging workforce:

> Managerial vision will necessarily encompass both philosophical and practical approaches to human resource management. A nonageist or age-neutral perspective will need to predominate. This will require a critical self-examination of both personal and corporate tendencies to age bias and stereotyping. (p. 18)

There are several key elements to this summary; we begin with managerial vision. The myths and stereotypes about aging workers are so ingrained, the practices that push them to obsolescence and marginalization so entrenched, that nothing less than the strongest commitment and follow-through of top management is necessary. It is first important that top management explicitly recognize the value of older workers and make a commitment to helping each older employee realize his or her full potential for productive work and broader contribution to the organization (Rosen & Jerdee, 1985). It is also important that management emphasize reasons other than legal compliance for this initiative, including the fact that better utilization of older employees makes good business sense and is socially responsible.

Walker (1999) has called for support not only from top management, but also from the human resources function; from unions, work councils, and professional associations; and from older employees themselves. It is important not to assume that older employees automatically buy into such initiatives; it is imperative therefore that their support be actively sought before initiation.

As Liebig (1988) noted, it is important to rid the organization of policies that are age-based. Hansson, DeKoekkoek, Neece, and Patterson (1997) also called for replacing those policies with others that specifically encourage the hiring and training of older workers. Straka (1998) called for an organization-wide emphasis on "continuous falsification and abandonment of chronological age as a valid criterion for decisions in human resource management" (p. 192). Probably far more policies and decisions are implicitly age-based than explicitly so (Marshall, 1998), and the implicit ones are difficult to detect and change. This highlights the need for organizational efforts to combat age stereotyping and age norms.

Combating Stereotypes and Age Norming

Liebig (1988) called for organizations to foster a "nonageist or age-neutral perspective" (p. 18). As noted earlier in this book, false and demeaning stereotypes of older workers are common. Indeed, they are the foundation for age discrimination and underutilization of older workers, and getting rid of them is an essential part of any organization's efforts to better use this population of workers.

Stereotypes are fallbacks that people use to make decisions when their perspective is biased or perhaps when they are simply too busy to devote sufficient thought to the unique characteristics of each person (Perry, Kulik, & Bourhis, 1996). They can have a profound impact on decision-making in areas such as hiring, training allocation, and performance management. Indeed, negative stereotypes become self-fulfilling prophecies. As an example of this, stereotypes of older workers as resistant to learning and change often result in denying them training opportunities and placing them in jobs that are not meaningful or cognitively challenging. As their skills become obsolete and their motivation declines, the stereotype is reinforced (Maurer, 2001).

Two closely related types of stereotyping behavior must be addressed. One is *age stereotypes* per se, which refer to implicit ideas people have about the relationship between age and worker characteristics. The other is *age norming of jobs and organizational contexts*, which essentially is implicit correlations between jobs or other organizational variables and the typical age of persons with which they are associated. For example, there is broad evidence in the literature that some jobs are seen as "older person" jobs and some are seen as "younger person" jobs (Finkelstein, Burke, & Raju, 1995). In addition, age norms can develop around organizational issues such as pay levels and duty assignments (Doeringer & Terkla, 1990). The problem with age norms is that they are generalizations that may bias decisions about specific individuals. In particular, an incongruence of circumstances with age can have a significant impact on evaluations. Age stereotyping and age norming distort evaluations of older workers and the decisions based on those evaluations. They suggest less variability in a group that is in fact becoming more variable with age. It is therefore imperative that organizations that seek to fully use older workers combat these distorting forces.

Changing long-held stereotypes is not an easy process. In part, it requires changing the perspectives and mechanisms on which age norms are based and age stereotypes operate. A useful first step may be an age audit (H. L. Sterns & Doverspike, 1988), where organizations investigate the distribution of age across jobs and how personnel decisions are differentially affecting persons by age. This may be useful, but it should also be emphasized that not all age differences are the result of stereotyping. Certainly, genuine differences in values and preferences exist among different age groups.

Beyond age audits, Perry et al. (1996) have recommended that organizations combat age norming by ensuring that older persons are more represented throughout the organization. This can be done through targeted recruitment and selection. Like Hale (1990), we recommend specific moves to make the contributions of older workers more visible and prominent throughout the organization.

Managerial Training

Training is an important tool in combating stereotypes and age norms and in helping to ensure a broader understanding of the older worker. We have noted throughout this book that the capabilities and needs of older workers are poorly understood, and the primary goal of managerial training for dealing with older workers is to help managers—especially younger managers (H. L. Sterns & Alexander, 1988; Tager, 1988)—better understand this group. However, as noted in Liebig's (1988) quote at the beginning of this section, a key role of this training is also to help managers understand themselves and, specifically, their age biases.

On the basis of our review of training recommendations offered in the literature and what is known about the special needs and challenges faced by older workers, we offer the following recommendations for the content of training courses for managers who deal with older workers. Many of these topics are important as well for training for younger co-workers and even for older workers themselves. Wineman (1988) has also emphasized the importance for unions and their membership to undergo such training. We urge broad-based training efforts to educate people on the special issues associated with the aging workforce.

Self-assessments of misconceptions and biases. As Hale (1990) noted, it is useful to include at the beginning of training a candid self-assessment of the misconceptions that people have about aging and older workers and the stereotypes and biases that have resulted. Deliberately confronting these entrenched ideas with facts in the course of the training program is a useful approach. For example, Perry et al. (1996) used a short measure of attitudes toward older workers that may be useful for such training self-assessments.

The aging process and its implications for the workplace. Training efforts must explore the myths and stereotypes as well as the life cycle changes that people go through as they age (Hale, 1990). It is an important task of training to identify myths, stereotypes, and age norms and to confront them not only with the realities of aging, but also the "snowballing" and self-fulfilling effects they have on older workers. Managers must be trained to recognize bias as well as the potential for bias and how to prevent it before it affects decisions (Liebig, 1988). As such, an accurate understanding of the characteristics of older workers and relationships between age and variables such as performance is essential. Presentation of the types, levels, and variability of changes that occur with aging can help them acquire a mind-set oriented less to age and more to functional capacity (Hale, 1990;

Warr, 1994). Dennis (1988b) noted that such programs should have an underlying philosophy of evaluating employees as individuals. In other words, all employees must be given equal opportunity to be successful, regardless of age. These programs should not be designed with the assumption that all older workers are competent or that only older workers should be employed. However, these programs should be based on an assumption that given comparable qualifications, older workers have the same potential and must be developed and supported in the same way that organizations invest in their younger employees.

Managers must understand the special needs of older workers and the situations that present difficulties for them. As an example, H. L. Sterns and Doverspike (1988) emphasized the important role that a manager can have in combating an older employee's reluctance to seek skill training. Managerial training may thus include an awareness of the barriers to retraining perceived by older workers, the myths and stereotypes that may influence training decisions for older workers, and means of cultivating a positive training environment for older employees and ensuring that training is given the priority it deserves.

Training on the special needs of older workers should include topics discussed later in this chapter and in chapter 8. For example, later in this chapter we present some principles associated with flexible work alternatives, and it is important that managers understand the need for such. Our presentations of training, performance management, and career management in the next chapter also contain much that managers should know.

Generational differences. Rosen and Jerdee (1985) have argued for training managers on the value differences between older and younger employees. They noted that the values of the older members of the workforce were shaped by the post-Depression period, World War II, and 1950s eras and may include a strong work ethic and an emphasis on job and financial security, family solidarity, respect for authority figures, and patriotism. Conversely, as Christensen (1990) suggested, younger members of the workforce grew up in homes that may have lacked traditional family structures and authority, and they may have a greater sense of entitlement and a weaker work ethic, place more value on leisure, and be more suspicious of authority figures and structures. Our aim here is not to suggest stereotypic views of different generations, but rather to point out that different generations have, in fact, been exposed to unique forces that have helped to shape them. Managers need to be aware of these generational differences.

H. L. Sterns and Alexander (1988), among others, have called attention to deeply held beliefs and attitudes that may make it especially difficult for younger persons to manage older ones. Younger managers may experience feelings of status conflict when supervising older employees, with their perceived status differences related to age—combined with a societal tendency to defer to the older—making it difficult to provide performance feedback and candidly deal with performance issues. In addition, younger managers who harbor stereotypes about the inability of older workers to change may avoid performance discussions with older workers. Finally, older workers may reject feedback out of a belief that the younger manager is inexperienced or impractical (Tager, 1988).

Training must address not only the existence of generational conflicts, but also ways and means for dealing with them. Rosen and Jerdee (1985) suggested that training should include discussion of generational differences and how they manifest themselves in work behavior; they should be exposed to a problem-solving process and trained to deal with the conflicts. They suggested the use of case studies, discussion of specific incidents, role-playing, and simulations to explore these differences. Additionally, Hale (1990) recommended training in listening skills and in conflict management, with a focus on generational conflicts between older and younger workers.

Knowledge of legal issues. Managers must understand the legal issues that pertain to the employment of older workers. Dennis (1988b), among others, has emphasized the importance of understanding discrimination law and the various prescriptions for managers that result from the law. Rosen and Jerdee (1985) emphasized the importance of thorough training for managers so that they can meet the difficult requirements of the Age Discrimination in Employment Act (ADEA).

Organizational Support Resources for Older Workers

Meeting the needs and desires of older workers requires that specific organizational support resources and mechanisms be designed with those needs in mind. Organizations should establish mechanisms for the reporting of age discrimination claims (Hale, 1990) and provide means by which they can be investigated and resolved short of litigation (Liebig, 1988). Career counseling programs that focus on long-term career management and flexible career and retirement alternatives not only help older workers but also help organizations to better use older workers, prevent obsolescence, and meet changing staffing needs. Hale noted the importance of programs to help older workers cope with life changes. These can be useful in the workplace, because the workplace can be a stabilizing influence in times of turbulent change.

Comprehensive preretirement programs are an essential part of this, and we discuss both career management and retirement programs in the next chapter. Hansson et al. (1997) noted the potential contributions of physical fitness and wellness programs, especially helpful for workers trying to overcome an intolerance to shift work that often develops at around age 40. Such programs also contribute to adjustment in retirement (Taylor & Doverspike, 2003).

Flexible Work Alternatives

Older employees continue to work for reasons other than the need for income and benefits. Indeed, it is often noted that in midlife workers begin to place more emphasis on intrinsic rewards from work, such as a feeling of accomplishment, of learning and experiencing new things, and of doing something worthwhile (Penner, Perun, & Steuerle, 2002). At the same time, however, older workers often go through a period of self-assessment that may lead them to place more emphasis on leisure and other nonwork pursuits (H. L. Sterns & Huyck, 2001) as well as question their willingness to tolerate stress in the workplace (A. A. Sterns, Sterns, & Hollis, 1996). The result is that they often want to continue working, but on different terms—with more flexible work arrangements, fewer hours, and jobs and work environments more responsive to their needs (Barth, McNaught, & Rizzi, 1995; Greller & Stroh, 2003; Shultz, 2003). Organizations have been slow to respond to these preferences and often maintain full-time work schedules in standard hierarchical positions up to the point of retirement. This has led many older workers to leave their career jobs earlier than they would like either to retire or for alternate work arrangements. This mismatch of work conditions with employee preferences causes needless upheaval in employees' lives and a critical loss to organizations of employee skill, experience, and savvy. Whereas the costs today often go unrecognized, in coming years labor shortages will convince organizations of the need to offer more flexible work alternatives.

Flexible work arrangements are in many ways mutually beneficial for older workers and employers. Alternatives such as allowing older workers to serve on temporary task forces or in temporary jobs allow them new opportunities for challenge and the development of new knowledge and skills (Farr et al., 1998). The AARP (2002) has stressed the value of such jobs in allowing employees to preview work environments and try out potential new jobs or lines of work. Through such arrangements organizations can reduce labor costs, gain staffing flexibility, reduce training costs (if employees who are already trained are used), gain more consistency in staffing over economic cycles, and retain valued workers. Finally, Paul (1988) observed that telecommuting and other work-at-home options may allow those with health or commuting issues to be productive, thus increasing the chances that organizations may retain the talents of these workers.

A variety of human resource management strategies have been suggested that offer older workers opportunities for (a) flexible work scheduling, (b) developing new knowledge and skills or using their current skills and abilities set differently, and (c) work environments tailored to their needs and preferences. A number of these strategies are discussed in the next sections.

Flexible Work Scheduling

Work-schedule adjustments may be a relatively simple method of keeping older workers motivated and productive. Many work-schedule innovations have already been used to address the needs of younger workers, especially in connection with child-care issues. Establishing such practices to respond to the wishes or needs of older workers may involve small additional monetary costs relative to the payoffs. In addition, innovative thinking about the "packaging" of work may be beneficial. For example, Robson (2001) described a flexible scheduling plan that redefines work in terms of 4-hour "work modules." Giving employees or managers the flexibility to set schedules in such units—long enough to allow completion of a reasonably large set of tasks but short enough to permit a variety of workdays and work weeks—might provide a good balance between completing tasks on time and offering flexibility in accommodating the needs of older and younger workers alike. Indeed, Sparks, Faragher, and Cooper (2001) noted that arrangements with flexible hours can result in lowered job stress, reduced absenteeism and tardiness, improved job satisfaction and productivity, and better work–family balance.

Job Sharing

Job sharing usually involves the splitting of one full-time job between two (or more) part-time workers. Rix (1990) noted that job sharing allows different skills, abilities, and perspectives to be brought to jobs; makes it easier for organizations to retain valued employees; provides a means for skill transfer from older to younger workers; and provides staffing continuity, because those sharing a job can fill in for each other as necessary.

Job Transfer and Special Assignments

Job transfers (especially if they are lateral transfers) allow workers to gain some variety in work activities, work with a different group of coworkers, and possibly even reduce the stressfulness of the work environment. They may include such temporary personnel activities as job rotation, where employees are allowed to move to different jobs with similar levels of responsibility. Some organizations assign older employees to special tasks that require a high level of organization-specific knowledge they have gathered over the years. These job placement practices can be an extremely useful way of using older workers, because they can be given assignments that match their particular interests and talents.

Beehr and Bowling (2002) noted that older workers may make excellent mentors for newer employees or serve as valuable advisors and sounding boards for decision makers in the organization. Many have noted the mutual value of such mentor–protégé relationships (e.g., Belous, 1990; Doeringer & Terkla, 1990; Marshall, 1998). Such relationships allow younger employees to benefit from the experience of older workers, and they provide older workers a means of staying involved and contributing. Certainly, moving older workers into mentoring roles puts them in a position where experience is valued. Not only does such an arrangement provide critical organizational knowledge transfer, but it can also be quite rewarding for the older workers.

Part-Time Work

An important key to offering an attractive workplace for older employees is to allow them to have choices through part-time or flexible working arrangements (Friedan, 1993; Hale, 1990; Wellner, 2002). Penner et al. (2002) cited surveys showing that 13% of those who had left the workforce or found other jobs after their career jobs would have stayed on with their career employer if they had been given the option to work fewer hours. Similarly, 19% of older workers working full time in 1998 said they would work fewer hours if offered. Similar results have been noted by Barth et al. (1995) and H. L. Sterns and Sterns (1995). However, Penner et al. cited surveys showing that few employees have the option of working fewer hours—in 1998, only 26% of employees ages 51 to 65 worked for employers that would allow reductions in hours. In addition, where organizations offer such an alternative, it is usually on a case-by-case basis rather than a program available to the broader group of older employees (Doeringer & Terkla, 1990).

Phased retirement. As noted in the previous chapter, phased retirement is a program that allows employees to gradually cut back on their work hours in order to "phase" into retirement. Penner et al. (2002) noted that phased retirement can be a very attractive option for older workers, although Greller and Stroh (2003) questioned whether such programs amount to anything more than a way to turn veteran employees into a contingent workforce.

Job and skills banks. A relatively recent innovation has been the creation of job banks for older workers, providing them with a variety of part-time employment opportunities. As described by Menchin (2000), these job banks can provide not only part-time work but also a diversity of assignments. Job banks are often established by companies as internal recruitment facilities for purposes of implementing flexible work arrangements for retirees and other experienced workers. Some companies refer to these temporary work pools as "skills banks" to note that they include high-responsibility positions requiring advanced engineering and technical skills. Job and skills banks help to offset the loss of valuable expertise that results from retirements and downsizing.

Bridge Jobs

Bridge employment is often part of the transitional process to retirement for older workers. Bridge jobs are jobs that one pursues after career employment is over to "bridge" the span between an attenuated career job and retirement. Doeringer (1990) noted that approximately one third of career jobs end by age 55 and almost half by age 60; because few retire at these ages, bridge employment for many workers may last a number of years. Indeed, today a majority of workers retire from bridge jobs rather than their career jobs (Shultz, 2003).

Bridge jobs quite often involve changes in occupation and industry, with significant losses in occupational status and pay (Christensen, 1990; Ruhm, 1990). Many bridge jobs are unskilled or are entry-level jobs generally filled by younger workers, with unattractive job content, poor working conditions, and poor job security (Doeringer & Terkla, 1990).

However, not all bridge jobs are so undesirable (Shultz, 2003). Higher quality bridge jobs are found in phased retirement programs of large corporations. They may also be found in informal arrangements by some firms to keep valued workers beyond the customary retirement age. As Doeringer (1990) noted, "these bridge jobs are often customized to the needs of individual workers. They provide the flexibility, economic benefits, and status that make bridge employment an attractive option to both career jobs and permanent retirement" (p. 12). Unlike the less desirable bridge jobs, these jobs preserve the match between worker competencies and job demands and thus allow more productive and fulfilling employment for older workers (Rebick, 1993; Shultz, 2003). Doeringer made the important point that these jobs are being created out of business necessity, not out of social consciousness. As the workforce ages, this business necessity will grow. Organizations will be forced to create attractive jobs with flexible arrangements to lure workers out of retirement.

Flexible work arrangements bring new challenges for organizations. Various issues including more difficult coordination and scheduling, and changes in the work culture have been noted (e.g., Sparks et al., 2001). Paul (1988) also warned that fringe benefit costs can be higher when spread over larger numbers of people, and unions may not be receptive to such arrangements (Applebaum & Gregory, 1990). Belous (1990) pointed out that temporary jobs often involve working with technology and that it may be difficult to recruit older employees for such jobs. Temporary agencies often make it easier for organizations to staff jobs with younger workers. However, as the workforce ages, organizations will need to find ways to address these challenges. As they do, flexible job arrangements will become more commonplace.

Flexible Compensation and Benefits

Evidence indicates that older workers have different preferences than younger workers in the areas of compensation and benefits (Hale, 1990). Whereas many older workers have a strong need for monetary compensation, benefits tend to become relatively more important to workers as they age (Belous, 1990). Older workers tend to choose different health care plans than younger workers, preferring fee-for-service plans to health maintenance organizations so that they have more flexibility in choosing providers

(Barringer & Mitchell, 1993). Wellner (2002) noted some compensation and benefits alternatives that may be palatable to older workers, including time off, schedule changes, and assistance in skill development in place of cash compensation. Workers can also work 80% time but be paid for 60%, with the rest going to fund health insurance.

Beyond preferences, compensation and benefits plans contain powerful incentives to work or not work. Most compensation and benefit plans in existence today are designed to encourage early exit from the workforce, both to reward long-term employees and get rid of higher cost workers without having to fire them (Penner et al., 2002). For example, defined benefit pension plans often contain incentives for retirement at around age 55 (Ekerdt, 1998).

Penner et al. (2002) noted the legal and regulatory difficulties for employers who wish to provide more flexible formal benefit plans to encourage older workers to continue working, and for workers who wish to work part-time. Requirements of uniformity built into the laws governing pensions and benefits make it all but impossible to set up separate formal programs for older employees. In addition, tax regulations require many pension recipients to quit working to receive benefits, thus depriving them of using their retirement benefits to supplement part-time employment. Penner et al. discussed various alternatives under existing laws that are beyond the scope of this book, but several points are noteworthy here. First, arrangements made on a case-by-case basis may not be problematic because they do not constitute a formal plan. Second, reduced hours or work schedules for current employees may not be problematic when offered to groups on the basis of length of service or job level rather than age. Third, for consultant or contractor relationships to be valid, the contracted employee must be able to set the conditions—how, when, and where—of work. If this condition is not met (and it may not be for many current "contractor" relationships), such persons may be considered employees rather than contractors, with possible tax penalties and retroactive benefits payments at stake. Penner et al. offered public policy suggestions to encourage flexible work and phased retirement, and it is our hope that legislators seriously consider these suggestions.

In general, organizations that wish to attract and retain older workers must be more flexible with compensation and benefits, just as they must be with work arrangements (Barringer & Mitchell, 1993). The specific needs and preferences of older workers must be addressed. Although such systems are challenging to establish, they are beneficial to both organizations and employees and worth considering.

Recruitment of Older Workers

Organizations may need to tailor their recruitment practices to attract older workers. For example, Belous (1990) has noted that traditional means of advertising jobs have had only limited success in recruiting older workers. Some of the more targeted techniques have included using older workers in the organization as part of the recruitment process and using parties and other social events to advertise pleasant working conditions.

Malatest (2003) suggested that a good strategy for finding older workers is by recruiting through more nontraditional channels such as journals, professional societies, and even posting notices in senior citizen centers. Rix (1990) reported that temporary agencies are useful sources to recruit older workers, as are the job banks found in certain industries that are especially labor-intensive or which require specialized skills. Belous (1990) also suggested that organizations tie wages and benefits together into a package to appeal to older workers' emphasis on benefits.

Little is currently known about recruiting older workers. For one, few organizations have made a systematic effort to do so, perhaps because they have not felt the need. In addition, we believe that the difficulties encountered are less those of marketing and salesmanship than of the product being sold—the overall attractiveness of jobs available to older workers. As we continue to better understand the needs of older workers, and as jobs and working conditions evolve to meet those needs, we expect that recruitment efforts will be better informed and more successful.

In the preceding pages we have described a number of organizational initiatives that represent the foundations of programs to use older workers. In order for these programs to be successful, the commitment must be there, policies must reflect the commitment, knowledge must be imparted and attitudes changed, support mechanisms must be in place, attractive alternatives must be offered, and older workers must be informed of them. We turn now from the foundations to the implementation of specific human resources programs for using older workers. We begin with matching persons to jobs where, once again, a new perspective is required.

Matching Persons to Jobs: Placement Issues

Our title for this section may imply the classical mechanisms of selection and placement. In light of an aging workforce and a looming prospect of labor shortages, a discussion of person–job matching takes a different focus from previous years. In the classic selection paradigm, organizations choose workers to fill positions on the basis of a match between worker characteristics and job requirements. The very use of the common term *job requirements* suggests that it is workers who are the changeable element; jobs are considered relatively static entities.

Economic and social forces will soon force a new paradigm. Although workers will still be matched to the requirements of jobs, job elements will become more variable entities than in the past. Rather than choosing workers with talents and interests that are the best match for the job, there will be more emphasis on changing jobs and working conditions to match the talents, preferences, and the developmental needs (Hall & Mirvis, 1995) of a fixed supply of workers. Placement will thus become a more prominent term than in the past, and one with an expanded meaning. Our discussion thus deals not only with selection and placement as typically understood, but with job design as well.

Selection

Any effort to select workers properly begins with a careful consideration of the challenges they must meet on the job. Job analyses are typically used to identify job requirements on which to base selection measures. Typical job analysis methods identify the tasks performed by workers and the knowledge, skills, and abilities required to perform those tasks. With the physical and psychological changes that occur with age, and especially with the variability of such changes, it is imperative to analyze jobs and compare them with the functional capacities of individual older workers (e.g., H. L. Sterns & Miklos, 1995; Warr, 1994). A. A. Sterns et al. (1996) advocated using job analytic techniques to identify the specific levels of task performance that are required on a job, so that those levels can be compared with individual capabilities. The comparison of job requirements to capabilities would be greatly served by psychological and physical attribute taxonomies to characterize jobs in a more fine-grained manner than job analytic methods often use (Faley, Kleiman, & Lengnick-Hall, 1984).

Although many of the descriptors in the abilities taxonomy of the O*NET occupational analysis system (Fleishman, Costanza, & Marshall-Mies, 1999) are at an appropriate level of specificity for this purpose, there still exists a need for standardized cognitive task analytic techniques for workplace tasks (Warr, 2001). Such techniques could assess work tasks for variables typically associated with age declines, such as working memory requirements and processing speed. Combined with similar benchmarks for assessing persons (for examples of physical ability and functional capacity assessments, see A. A. Sterns et al., 1996), such techniques could allow older workers to be assessed for fit to a job and vice versa. This emphasis on assessment of individual functional capacity is consistent with the requirements of the Americans With Disabilities Act (A. A. Sterns et al., 1996).

As noted earlier in this book, older workers can often compensate in their performance for age-related declines in certain capacities. For example, older workers develop work strategies that can compensate for their loss of information-processing efficiency (cf. Fisk & Rogers, 2000; Schooler et al., 1998). This adds a layer of challenge to task-analytic techniques and selection. It suggests, as Hoyer (1998) recommended, the use of high-fidelity job simulations wherever possible in selection, because such measures allow compensating mechanisms to influence test performance. Also, as Farr et al. (1998) suggested, given the demonstrated association between job knowledge and job performance and the wealth of work experience that older workers often have accumulated, it makes sense to emphasize knowledge in selection and placement decisions.

There is a need to learn more about the impact of age on the mean score levels, construct validity, and criterion-related validity of personnel selection measures. One might expect older persons to be at a disadvantage on highly speeded tests, and the use of these measures should only be considered when the job in question requires such speed. On measures that are not speeded, older persons typically perform as well as younger ones (Sonnenfeld, 1988); indeed, on measures such as job knowledge or other experiential assessments, older experienced persons may have an advantage (Warr, 2001).

Likewise, measures of physical ability may put older workers at a disadvantage. Once again, it is important to match carefully the physical ability level sought to the level required in the job. As noted earlier in this book, the existence of an age-related decline, either physical or psychological, does not necessarily place a person below the threshold necessary for job performance (Schooler et al., 1998).

Selection measures that require human judgment in the scoring processes (e.g., structured interviews, assessment exercises) are susceptible to the age-stereotyping and age-norming effects mentioned earlier. It is therefore important that evaluators be properly trained. Our suggestions in the next chapter for performance evaluation procedures and training of raters are generally applicable to judgment-based selection evaluations as well.

When testing older persons, the testing medium should be carefully considered. The most obvious concern here is the use of computer-based tests, which may place older persons at a disadvantage if they have not been given opportunities to become familiar with such equipment and to practice using it (Johnson & White, 1980; Walker, 1999).

It is reasonable to assume that selection and placement efforts for older workers will make more use of worker preferences than has often been the case as organizations focus more than they had in the past on the appeal of work to draw older workers to the workplace. Issues such as location of work and work hours will become more salient in selection and placement efforts. We also believe that organizations will put more emphasis on what has classically been known as *placement* to find those jobs in the organization to which older workers are best suited. For example, Farr et al. (1998) observed that older workers' strengths are often found in areas of organizational citizenship, such as assistance to others with work or personal problems, organizational support roles, orienting new employees, and the like. They also noted that older workers tend to be well suited to jobs such as customer service, jobs where conscientiousness and attention to detail are emphasized, and jobs that involve quality control and continuous quality improvements.

Job Design

As noted earlier in this chapter, we believe that jobs will be increasingly redesigned to accommodate the effects of aging as well as to make them more appealing to workers so that they stay in or return to the workforce. Areas for redesign suggested by the aging literature may be as diverse as work location, job content, work pacing, autonomy for completing assigned tasks, the physical environment, tools and work aids, and so on (e.g., Hansson et al., 1997; Warr, 2001). Flexible work alternatives may also be considered job redesign because they alter the basic working conditions of the job.

Job redesign can sometimes be an expensive process (Hale, 1990; Paul, 1988), and organizations have tended to do it on a case-by-case basis rather than offer systematic programs (Rix, 1990). However, job redesign has several potential benefits for organizations beyond better use of older workers. First, it allows organizations to retain valued workers. Second, it can increase the productivity and satisfaction of workers. Third, ergonomically redesigned workplaces can make jobs safer for all employees (H. L. Sterns & Miklos, 1995). Finally, Faley et al. (1984) noted that job redesign may be critical in preventing legal action under the ADEA. That job redesign may have extra payoffs for older workers is suggested by research reported by Hansson et al. (1997), who noted that poor tool design had more negative effects on the work performance of older workers than younger workers.

Job redesign can be as idiosyncratic as the jobs themselves and the people who occupy them. Some major categories of job redesign for older workers include the following:

1. *Physical redesign.* Ergonomic workplace design can reduce the potential for strain and injury (Farr et al., 1998). For example, special supports can be used for workers who must stand all day (Paul, 1988), and supports can be used to reduce the need for bending, stretching, or lifting (A. A. Sterns et al., 1996; Warr, 2001). A. A. Sterns et al. (1996) noted the need for custom workstation design to match older employees' body structures and sensory capabilities. For example, computer workstations of older employees should have monitors with adjustable height so that older workers wearing bifocals or trifocals do not have to strain to see them.

2. *Sensory redesign.* To compensate for losses of sensory skills, jobs can be redesigned with improvements such as larger computer screens, larger print on warning signs, better lighting, use of easily discriminated colors, and sound amplification (Faley et al., 1984; Hansson et al., 1997; A. A. Sterns et al., 1996; Warr, 2001).

3. *Information processing redesign.* Warr (1994) observed that declines in information-processing ability make it more difficult for older persons to rely on internal representations of information. To accommodate this, jobs can be redesigned with decision-making aids such as flowcharts, written procedures, lists, menus for action, and so on. One key potential use of technology with older employees is the use of computers to handle routine information processing so that older employees' cognitive resources can be freed to bring more knowledge and experience to tasks.

4. *Work flow and pace redesign.* Older workers may function better with a slower work pace or one that they control (M. L. Levine, 1988) as a means of avoiding fatigue (Czaja & Sharit, 1993; Hale, 1990). For example, A. A. Sterns et al. (1996) advocated periods of rest between episodes of physical exertion.

5. *Redesign for stress control.* A. A. Sterns et al. (1996) noted the importance of removing stressors from work environments, because such stressors can be more distracting for

older workers. These include factors such as information overload, noise, overcrowding, dirt, and poor air quality.

Conclusion

In this chapter, we have discussed areas of concern for organizations that wish to better utilize older workers. We noted some important organizational requirements, including a strong commitment by top management, age-neutral policies, efforts to combat age stereotyping and age norming, managerial training, and support resources for older employees. We also discussed several organizational strategies, including flexible work alternatives, flexible compensation and benefits, and targeted recruitment that may attract older workers. Finally, we discussed the processes of placing older workers in jobs, emphasizing the complementary processes of selection–placement and job redesign.

So far, we have dealt with the processes that bring older workers to organizations and potentially effective work environments. In the next chapter, we turn to the mechanisms for ensuring ongoing performance, including training, performance appraisal, and career development.

Chapter

8

Training, Performance Management, and Career Management

In the previous chapter, we considered the processes necessary to establish an organization that can fully utilize older workers as well as the placement of those workers in jobs. In this chapter, we discuss several additional important processes. Training is important not only for initial job placement but also for combating obsolescence over the long term. Our discussion includes several types of formal and informal training, and we present principles for the effective training of older workers. Performance appraisal is an essential part of any organization's effort to ensure a productive workforce. We discuss the role of performance appraisal and offer suggestions for its implementation with an older workforce. Career development and retirement are often thought of as largely individual processes, but we show that organizations have important stakes in them as well.

Training

One of the most persistent stereotypes of older workers is that they are not worth training. Studies have shown that older workers are consistently viewed as untrainable, not interested in training, and a poor place to invest training resources because of their attenuated careers (e.g., Novelli, 2002). As a result, older workers are often denied training opportunities (Farr, Tesluk, & Klein,

1998), their skills degrade and become obsolete, and, once again, the perception becomes a self-fulfilling prophecy. It is imperative that organizations ensure equal access to training for older workers, in part because not doing so is a violation of the Age Discrimination in Employment Act (ADEA; H. L. Sterns, 1986).

A meta-analysis of training studies by Kubeck, Delp, Haslett, and McDaniel (1996) showed that compared with younger workers, older workers tend to show less mastery of training material, take longer to learn the tasks being taught, and take longer to complete training programs. Generalizing from these observations to the above stereotypes is a considerable leap, however. The general idea that older employees are less trainable has been challenged (e.g., H. L. Sterns & Doverspike, 1988); Warr (1994) stated that "the factors limiting their learning primarily concern expectations and corporate norms rather than major deficits in information processing abilities" (p. 536). In addition, Kubeck et al. pointed out that the posttraining differences observed between older and younger trainees may be a function of pretraining levels and thus may not necessarily mean that older trainees receive less benefit from training.

A growing literature suggests that, in fact, the differences attributed to age may be due at least in part to factors external to older workers. Training is rarely tailored to the learning skills or the interests of older adults. Indeed, typical organizational training environments are often poor learning environments for older adults (Schooler, Caplan, & Oates, 1998). We believe this is also a contributing explanation for the results of Kubeck et al. (1996), and later in this section we discuss training principles tailored to older workers. It may also explain why older employees are often hesitant to participate in training (H. L. Sterns & Doverspike, 1988). Indeed, D. A. Peterson and Wendt (1995) cited survey results showing that a significant number of older employees do not take advantage of training opportunities because they believe that the training would not help in their job and that instructors would not be sensitive to their needs.

Some surveys and studies have shown that older employees are interested in training (Hale, 1990); Simpson, Geller, and Stroh (2002) reported a high level of training activity among older workers in response to recent competitive pressures in the labor market. Simpson et al. criticized studies showing a lower participation in training among older employees, because such studies typically focus only on employer-provided training. They observed that older workers are actually more likely to participate in training off the job, a result reinforced by survey results cited by D. A. Peterson and Wendt (1995). Simpson et al. demonstrated in their study that younger workers are more likely to seek apprenticeships and training in basic skills. Older employees are more likely to invest in training that is directly job related, including credentialing programs, targeted career and job-related courses, and on-the-job computer-based training. Warr (2001) also noted higher interest among older workers in training that is directly job related. The low interest level of older workers for many in-house training programs may say more about the content of those programs, their job relevance, and the degree of comfort they afford older trainees than it does about older workers' general interest in training.

There is also the issue of whether training investments in older workers are recovered given the shorter time left in their careers. As noted in chapter 6, older workers have less job turnover than younger employees (Rhodes, 1983); thus, in many cases, training investments are more likely to be recovered with older workers (Rix, 1990).

Nevertheless, that older employees tend to realize a lower level of training mastery, and take longer to do so than younger employees, is a persistent finding separate from the Kubeck et al. (1996) meta-analysis (e.g., Forteza & Prieto, 1994; Hoyer, 1998; Rix, 1990; Schooler et al., 1998; H. L. Sterns & Doverspike, 1988; Warr, 1994, 2001). A growing literature suggests, however, that the differences attributable to age may be due in significant part to factors external to older workers and that training difficulties can be surmounted at least to some extent by proper training design and by giving attention to the training environment.

Training Principles for Older Workers

Effective training principles for older workers must recognize their unique situation. Their information-processing abilities may have declined such that they are no longer able to learn new material as efficiently as they once did, and they are more susceptible to distraction (e.g., Sonnenfeld, 1988). However, older workers often have the benefits of more knowledge and experience on which to link new training (Warr, 2001). They may falsely attribute their training difficulties to an inability to retain information (Hansson et al., 1997) and thus lose confidence in their ability to profit from training (Warr, 1994). Their confidence may be further eroded by being overlooked for training and by past experiences with training that may have been poorly designed for them (Farr et al., 1998). They may have more fear of failure in training and fear of embarrassment, especially in the presence of younger trainees, in part because their previous training experiences may have been some time ago.

Researchers have discussed a wide variety of training strategies that have been shown to be useful in training older adults. Research has demonstrated that these principles will also enhance younger adult performance; that is, better training for older adults is better training for all workers. Below, we provide a description of some of the more salient training principles. These principles reflect what we know about cognitive and physical changes with aging, preferences of older workers, and the importance of individual factors such as self-efficacy to training.

Conduct outreach. Given the frequent detachment of older employees from training, it is important to ensure that learning opportunities, and the benefits of pursuing them for older workers, are well publicized (Straka, 1998). Likewise, older workers need to be proactive in searching for and pursuing opportunities (Rix, 1990).

Attend to motivation and confidence. H. L. Sterns (1986) noted that older trainees often enter training with a fear of failure and a poor sense of self-efficacy. Trainers must help them put aside past negative experiences, encourage them throughout the program, and provide ample positive feedback. Training should be structured to provide early, reinforcing successes. It is also recommended that training programs address the rewards that stem from mastery and completion of training and tie these rewards to issues important to older workers (Hale, 1990).

Train in strategies for effective learning. Warr (1994) noted that older learners may need help "relearning how to learn"

(p. 535), because many have been away from training for a long time. Training in learning strategies (e.g., rehearsal strategies, using memory aids, utilizing organization) and issues such as time management and anxiety reduction can be useful (H. L. Sterns & Doverspike, 1988).

Use clearly relevant training. We have already discussed the preference of older workers for training content that is clearly and directly job-related and practical, rather than theoretical or basic skill-related (Hale, 1990; H. L. Sterns & Miklos, 1995). H. L. Sterns and Doverspike (1988) also emphasized the importance of similarity between the training and job environments for transfer. Wellner (2002) suggested allowing older workers to help design the training in order to ensure its relevance.

Emphasize the concrete over the abstract. Older learners may grasp concrete concepts more readily than abstract ones (Warr, 1994, 2001). If abstract material is required, trainers should explain the rationale and how the abstract knowledge is needed to perform specific tasks on the job (Rix, 1990).

Incorporate procedural performance in instruction where possible. Fisk and Rogers (2000) also showed that training of older persons can be enhanced by using action-based training that uses procedural performance rather than simply concept-based, declarative learning. They noted that this principle has been used with success in training older persons to use automatic teller machines, conduct online searches, and use the Internet.

Use active and open learning. Older persons are often many years removed from classrooms, so classroom-oriented training can be anxiety provoking and uninteresting to them. Hale (1990) suggested actively involving older learners in the training process through case studies, simulations or exercises, role-plays, and other participative means (see also Fisk & Rogers, 2000). She also noted the importance of providing ample opportunities for questions and discussion. Small group learning can also be effective (Fisk & Rogers, 2000; Warr, 1994). Forteza and Prieto (1994) and H. L. Sterns (1986) argued for the use of discovery learning where learners actively develop principles and relationships largely on their own, but with guided assistance from trainers. Similarly, Rix (1990) and H. L. Sterns (1986) advocated experiential learning. Czaja (1996) demonstrated success with computer-based training by structuring it into a series of problem-solving exercises. Training should also offer self-study resources that older persons can consult as needed (Fisk & Rogers, 2000; Warr, 2001).

Incorporate modeling using older workers. Maurer (2001) noted that self-efficacy is improved when people observe persons similar to themselves succeeding. Therefore, training can be enhanced by using older persons as actors in training materials and as trainers and facilitators. Warr (2001) advocated visible recognition of training achievements by older persons and encouragement in training from older role models.

Attend to the sensory and physical environment. Training environments for older workers may require larger print, better lighting, and clearer enunciation of content than those for younger workers. Distractions should be minimized. In addition, some older workers may find it difficult to stand or sit for extended periods, so frequent breaks should be provided (Forteza & Prieto, 1994).

Ensure transfer to and reinforcement on the job. H. L. Sterns and Doverspike (1988) and Warr (2001) noted the importance of manager and peer encouragement and reinforcement of training in the job setting. They observed that relapse prevention techniques and goal setting can be used to ensure that training is incorporated into the job environment.

Good instructional design depends on careful needs analysis, and evaluation of training is essential as well. Our presentation has focused on elements that are especially important for older learners, but more general principles of effective instruction are also relevant. Finally, it is important to address practical barriers, such as expense or a lack of transportation, that are often salient for older workers and that prevent them from taking advantage of training (Peterson & Wendt, 1995).

Technology Training

The common observations that older learners have difficulty learning and take longer to do so are also prevalent in technology training (cf. Czaja, 1996; Czaja & Sharit, 1993). B. Goldberg (2000) noted, however, that survey trends suggest that older workers are becoming more comfortable with new technology. Not surprisingly, this parallels the retirement of workers with less experience using computers. If this trend continues, older workers should continue to express more and more comfort with technology, which should ease the training challenge. In any event, the principles for effective technology training are essentially the same as the effective training principles noted above. The training of older workers on computer technology is extremely valuable for a number of reasons. Many jobs in our economy require computer skills, and many older persons are currently reluctant to take such jobs (Belous, 1990). In addition, as noted in chapter 7, jobs could be designed to allow computers to perform routine information processing tasks that may tax the cognitive resources of older workers (Warr, 2001). Beyond the work setting, however, technology training has the potential to greatly enhance the quality of life and independence of older persons. Czaja (1996) has discussed a number of ways in which this is possible. For example, computers allow more home-based employment opportunities, especially for those who have health or transportation impediments. Facility with computers can also result in more access to training and more opportunities to increase knowledge and skill.

Combating Obsolescence

The pace of change in our economy makes competence rather perishable. A number of authors (e.g., Dubin, 1990; Farr et al., 1998, Rosen & Jerdee, 1985) have written of the disturbingly short half-life of competence in highly technical jobs—as short as 1 to 2 years in fields such as computers and engineering. Performance in many jobs peaks at an early age; Howard (1998) observed that employees in some professional and technical jobs peak as early as their 20s or 30s. Skill and knowledge obsolescence is indeed a major challenge in our economy, not only because of the pace of change but also because of increased demand for professional accountability and the pressures of global competition (Dubin, 1990).

Our society devotes a great deal of effort to teaching competence but is neither effective nor efficient at refreshing it. A survey reported by H. L. Sterns and Miklos (1995) showed that only 23% of organizations have programs to combat obsolescence.

Because change has accelerated over the past few decades at the same time that the labor pool has expanded, organizations have tended to regard workers as depreciable—or, in some cases, disposable—assets (Rosen & Jerdee, 1985). This has taken a toll on organizational productivity, worker well-being, and the performance of our economy. Obsolescence is a phenomenon that is often ignored for long periods by both organizations and workers, and by the time it is noticed, it is often difficult to address. For example, by the time it becomes clear that some workers need retraining, they may have family obligations that make it impractical for them to leave the workforce for the time it takes for such retraining (Rosen & Jerdee, 1985).

Older workers are often hit the hardest by obsolescence. Not only is their training often more out of date, but they may also be victims of age stereotypes that result in them being denied opportunities to reverse the obsolescence—thus resulting in a self-fulfilling prophecy of obsolescence being associated with, and attributed to, age (Friedan, 1993).

Combating obsolescence requires individual effort and organizational encouragement (Dubin, 1990). On an individual level, employees must take responsibility for managing their careers and their own continuous development. On an organizational level, there are many measures that can be taken to encourage and facilitate continuous updating of skills. Some mentioned by Dubin (1990), Kaufman (1990), and D. B. Miller (1990) include a strong commitment by management to training and development and the improvement of performance, directing resources to training and coaching and allowing employees time to pursue such opportunities, fostering an environment that rewards innovation and technical excellence, incorporating skill maintenance as an important component of the performance appraisal system, and using challenging work assignments and job rotation to challenge employees. Farr and Middlebrooks (1990) pointed out that many organizations simply remove some constraints from development (e.g., by reimbursing for tuition) but do not address positive incentives for pursuing it. They emphasized the importance of the organization explicitly rewarding learning goals as well as performance goals in order to maintain and enhance technical competence. H. L. Sterns and Huyck (2001) noted that organizations that emphasize skill maintenance and development while also providing challenging work and the opportunity to innovate are rewarded through a more capable workforce, less turnover, and increased competitive advantage.

With the aging of the workforce, worker shortages may result in more organizations coming to regard employees as renewable assets. Some organizations are already discovering the benefits of doing so. Rosen and Jerdee (1985) reported that General Electric estimated the cost of retraining engineers at one third the cost of replacing them. It is important that both older workers and organizations take measures to fight obsolescence of workers' skills. As in many things, the best approach seems to be an incremental and continuous one. For example, H. L. Sterns and Doverspike (1988) stated that lifelong retraining is useful because workers can later build on previous knowledge and experience.

A variety of ongoing approaches are available for refreshing skills and keeping employees motivated. Dubin (1990) and Hall and Mirvis (1995) argued for novelty in assignments and experiences to challenge workers. In-house interventions such as job rotations, short-term assignments (task forces, project teams, etc.), coaching and feedback, and continuous learning through on-the-job problem solving can be used for many workers. Formal retraining is also useful. For scientific or technical personnel, involvement in in-service training, professional meetings, classes, or paid sabbaticals can be effective. For management personnel, continuing education, in-house workshops, and intensive in-house training with case studies and computer simulations have also been advocated (Rosen & Jerdee, 1985).

Robson (2001) noted that the pace of technological change and its effect on the workforce make training a natural preoccupation for organizations contemplating an aging workforce. Changes in average education levels of aging workers may make this challenge easier to deal with than is often assumed, and older workers themselves represent a training resource that is often insufficiently tapped. For individuals who are already employed, the fast pace of change and the rate at which technology has rendered many jobs obsolete have made the need for lifelong learning obvious. In fact, Hall and Mirvis (1995), in discussing continuous learning as a developmental strategy for older workers, suggested that the focus of training should be on when the learning is demanded by the job.

Continuous learning and skill development by workers of all ages is becoming more important than ever before. Maurer (2001) noted that although mid- and late-career stages used to be viewed as periods of mastery and maintenance (with no real demand for learning new things), now all workers are increasingly being called on to continuously learn and adapt. Indeed, new skills are required of workers at midlife and beyond just to continue to perform their jobs, and those who do not embrace the notion of continuous learning may find their careers cut short (Greller & Stroh, 1995).

One final point about obsolescence is relevant: Organizations must monitor for obsolescence and control it (Kaufman, 1990). Rosen and Jerdee (1985) and Kaufman advocated the use of surveys of training needs, administered to both management and nonmanagement employees. Another approach is to use performance appraisal data to identify worker retraining needs and incorporate retraining objectives as part of the performance management process (Dubin, 1990). We now turn to performance management principles associated with the aging workforce.

Performance Management

Performance appraisal and management systems are essential for the proper use of all human resources, not just older workers. Personnel decisions such as promotions, compensation, training, and layoff or termination must be based on accurate performance information. Performance information is critical as well for workers who want to improve their job performance (H. L. Sterns & Alexander, 1988).

With older workers, a performance appraisal system can contribute to removing the explicit or implicit emphasis on age as a basis for decisions. Older workers who are able to meet work objectives can be identified and retained, and those who cannot might be retrained or counseled to leave the organization (Warr, 1994). Under the ADEA, personnel decisions are far more defensible when based on a "systematic, objective, and job-related performance appraisal system" (Rosen & Jerdee, 1985, p. 74). Indeed, C. S. Miller, Kaspin, and Schuster (1990) found that the existence of a performance appraisal system as the basis for promotion and demotion was very convincing to courts in ADEA cases. Organizations cannot simply rest on assumptions that performance declines with age (H. L. Sterns & Miklos, 1995).

The basic characteristics of a performance appraisal system for older workers are really no different than those for younger workers. For most jobs, the system will be at least partially based on subjective rating criteria. The system must be aligned with the strategic goals of the organization, and the organization must further place priority on conducting accurate and timely reviews of performance (Rosen & Jerdee, 1985). The rating criteria must represent job-related constructs shown in a job analysis to have demonstrable relationships to organizational effectiveness, and they must be comprehensive as a set so that no important areas of performance are left out. The rating procedure must clearly differentiate levels of effectiveness in specific, behavioral terms (Barrett & Kernan, 1987). Overall, the system must be legally defensible so that the judgments that result can be considered accurate reflections of actual performance. The system must also be administratively feasible (Rosen & Jerdee, 1985; H. L. Sterns & Alexander, 1988).

The persons conducting such appraisals must be qualified and have sufficient exposure to the ratee's job performance to make accurate assessments. Raters may be supervisors or some combination of supervisors, peers, subordinates, and even customers. However, some have advocated that all persons providing ratings of older employees be trained to prevent age bias (H. L. Sterns & Miklos, 1995). Perry, Kulik, and Bourhis (1996) found that age bias is a measurable characteristic that seems to predispose some to see older persons in a more negative light and to more easily incorporate age stereotypes and age norms in evaluations. Similar to the managerial training discussed in the previous chapter, rater training should include an assessment of participants' attitudes and beliefs at the beginning of training, an exploration of the myths versus realities of aging, and the dangers of inferring characteristics of individuals from age stereotypes and age norms of jobs and work situations. In essence, the idea is to train raters to ensure that performance evaluations are based on the unique performance of each individual rather than on group membership or group stereotypes (Hansson, DeKoekkoek, Neece, & Patterson, 1997).

Research has related various situational, ratee, and rater characteristics in an attempt to learn the conditions under which age bias is more salient. Overall, results of this research have been inconsistent and difficult to interpret (Finkelstein, Burke, & Raju, 1995). However, we offer some generalizations that seem appropriate. One is to differentiate the older ratee from the group stereotype to the greatest extent possible by ensuring that ample specific performance information is available for each individual rated. Another is to avoid, where possible, comparing older and younger ratees, so that attention is not drawn to the age difference (Finkelstein et al., 1995). Finally, the importance of the rating task should be emphasized, sufficient time should be given to completing ratings, and distractions should be minimized. In addition, a control system in which the impact of ratings is assessed (H. L. Sterns & Alexander, 1988) and ratings are reviewed can motivate raters to provide the needed attention to the rating task.

Reviews of court cases dealing with performance appraisals yield some additional suggestions for performance appraisal and management systems. Barrett and Kernan (1987) found that courts look most favorably on systems that (a) apply standards equally to all employees, (b) incorporate a review by upper management to prevent biased results from individual managers, and (c) supplement appraisals with performance counseling to address inadequate performance. In their review of ADEA cases, C. S. Miller, Kaspin, and Schuster (1990) found that courts expect performance appraisals to be credible and fair. Miller et al. also observed that when performance appraisals are used as the basis for layoffs, the courts tend to look favorably on a type of system that "breaks ties" in favor of older employees.

The accurate assessment of performance is a key tool for organizations that wish to fully use older workers. Not only are such assessments important for making decisions about employees, they also allow older employees to develop when the performance management system includes discussion of performance issues and mutual goal-setting (Rosen & Jerdee, 1985). We turn now to longer term issues in career development of older workers.

Career Management

The classic idea of a career has been working full time in a primary occupation, often for one employer, until retirement. Much of the body of knowledge in vocational counseling is based on this model (H. L. Sterns & Miklos, 1995). However, the competitive pressures of the global economy, the switch from a manufacturing to a service-based economy, the rapid pace of technological change, and changing social systems have combined to redefine the career model into a more discontinuous one. This new career model generally involves working in multiple occupations, for multiple organizations, and in a more competitive job market. Furthermore, career success is being redefined to mean adaptability and mobility across occupations and organizations rather than upward mobility within an organization (e.g., Howard, 1998; H. L. Sterns, 1998). Careers are no longer measured by life spans of people but by life spans of competencies (Hall & Mirvis, 1995).

The free-agency model in sports is fast becoming a model for the larger economy (H. L. Sterns & Gray, 1999; H. L. Sterns & Kaplan, 2003), and it might be said that careers no longer belong to organizations, but to individuals. As such, workers now must manage their own careers. Career self-management requires a new strategic focus on self-directed and continuous learning of new skill sets and adaptability to change (Doeringer, 1990; Farr et al., 1998; Hall & Mirvis, 1995; Hansson et al., 1997). Careers are becoming highly individualized, shaped by idiosyncratic needs and values, with a goal of individual fulfillment rather than external success. Self-directed career management will thus blur the distinction between work and nonwork, incorporating not only work-related aspirations but also desires for leisure and nonwork activities.

H. L. Sterns and his colleagues (H. L. Sterns & Gray, 1999; H. L. Sterns & Kaplan, 2003) argued that the forces responsible for vesting career responsibility with the individual may have a disproportionate impact on older workers. Downsizing and restructuring and the attendant career instability may be more salient for older workers because they are often the victims of stereotypes about retraining and career viability. In addition, they often occupy the middle management positions that are most affected by organizational cuts. However, H. L. Sterns and colleagues also noted that the new emphasis on career self-management may work to the advantage of older workers, leading them to be valued more for their knowledge and experience.

H. L. Sterns and his colleagues (H. L. Sterns & Gray, 1999; H. L. Sterns & Kaplan, 2003) noted that career self-management requires a level of responsibility for which some individuals are not prepared. Although the responsibility for career management is coming to rest more with individual workers, organizations have a strong interest in assisting with the process, because better career self-management can lead to less obsolescence and more motivated and satisfied workers.

Organizations can assist with the process by providing career management resources to all employees. Doing so would provide workers with additional information and assistance that can be very beneficial in dealing with the rapidly changing employment market. From an organizational viewpoint, strategic career management programs based on careful human resource (HR) planning can help organizations keep valued employees, especially older ones; fill positions that may be difficult to adequately fill from the external market because of the specialized training, knowledge, or expertise involved (Hale, 1990); and reduce personnel costs through retraining existing workers rather than hiring new ones (Rosen & Jerdee, 1985). With careful foresight, career management functions can help organizations adapt more nimbly to changing circumstances by retaining accumulated expertise and experience while continuously refreshing skills.

Both Hale (1990) and Rosen and Jerdee (1985) have proposed career development models, with Hale's being from a more individual perspective and Rosen and Jerdee's from a more organizational one. Hale emphasized the importance of exploring the current versus desired capabilities, preferences, and motivations of individual workers and developing strategies for moving from the current to the desired state. Rosen and Jerdee's model includes an assessment of organizational strategic plans for their HR implications; projection of work capabilities needed to meet the strategic goals; analysis of the characteristics of existing employees (their past performance, their current knowledge and skill sets, aspirations, constraints, etc.); analysis of opportunities and constraints from the external environment that may affect recruitment, selection, and training; and development and implementation of a plan to effect the match between strategic plans and workforce capabilities. Essentially, the capabilities of the existing workforce—through proactive means rather than the accidental ones that govern many organizations—come to be aligned with strategic plans, and continuous learning and adaptability prepare the workforce for contingencies that strategic plans cannot always anticipate. The HR plan to ensure the match between strategic plans and workforce capabilities should include tools discussed in this chapter and in the previous one to allow the participation of older workers.

Computerized systems are critical tools for accomplishing this task in medium-sized to larger organizations (Farr et al., 1998; Hall & Mirvis, 1995; H. L. Sterns & Doverspike, 1988). Such systems can characterize the existing workforce, match it to job demands, and assess mismatches as an aid to HR planning. They can also identify linkages between demands of different jobs that can be useful in making transfer and promotion decisions, with an emphasis on both performance and growth. They can facilitate self-assessments of workers and better communicate job opportunities.

In career counseling with older workers, the stresses brought on by the changing career must be addressed. Hansson et al. (1997) noted the need to develop "occupational self-efficacy" in older workers by enhancing their beliefs in their relevance to changing organizational goals, their ability to be productive, their capability to change and to learn new technologies, and their social competence in the organization. Canaff (1997) noted some unique issues that arise in career counseling with older workers: They may not believe that seeking help is an accepted behavior, they may find change more challenging, and career counseling (much more so than with younger workers) tends to touch all facets of their lives. For older workers who must investigate new jobs, Canaff noted the need to assist them with job search and with issues such as resume writing and interview skills, because their experience with these may be dated.

H. L. Sterns and Patchett (1984) suggested that transitions in work life may occur many times in the course of a career. Indeed, many older adults are interested in working past traditional retirement age and further developing their careers and even possibly changing jobs. This new focus on employment opportunities with late career employees has also begun to change the way retirement planning is viewed.

Retirement Planning

Just as careers are changing, so is retirement. Previously viewed as a relatively discrete, point-in-time phenomenon at the end of career employment, retirement is being recognized as a more gradual process that can unfold over a longer period of time (Ekerdt, 1998), with perhaps multiple exits from and entries into the workforce. It is also a process that places a great deal of importance on adjustment, with far-reaching implications for all parts of life (Forteza & Prieto, 1994; Friedan, 1993).

Retirement planning plays a pivotal role in adjustment to retirement. Taylor and Doverspike (2003) reviewed research showing that retirement planning can be linked to lower anxiety and depression, better attitudes toward retirement, better postretirement adjustment, and workforce exit at an earlier age. They believe that these effects are primarily related to the "formation of realistic expectations about the social and financial aspects of retirement" (p. 59). In addition, the planning process facilitates the setting of goals for financial, physical, and social well-being after retirement, with the goals leading to more planning and preparatory activity.

Retirement planning programs are becoming more popular in organizations (H. L. Sterns & Miklos, 1995), in part to promote retirement (Dennis, 1988c). They are also becoming more encompassing in scope, moving from primarily financial to covering more of the social and psychological issues of retirement (H. L. Sterns & Doverspike, 1988). Some of the issues being addressed in programs include financial planning, health and wellness issues, living arrangements, use of time, interpersonal relationships, caring for older parents, and substance abuse (Dennis, 1988c; Forteza & Prieto, 1994). Retirement programs have also begun to deal with employment and career development topics, as employment during retirement is common and will become more common as labor force changes unfold in the near future.

Dennis (1988c) advocated the need for retirement planning programs to emphasize role change; psychological and social impacts of leaving the workforce; and specialized needs associated with health, socioeconomic status, and gender and minority status. She also advocated offering retirement planning programs earlier, because many participants noted that they wish they had started this planning earlier.

Taylor and Doverspike (2003) suggested that retirement planning programs focus on building self-efficacy to meet the challenges and changes in retirement and reducing the ambiguity and uncertainty of the retirement process. Noting that better health leads to higher levels of adjustment and satisfaction in retirement, they argued for "a frank discussion of the importance of physical well-being on subsequent adjustment" (p. 63), along with instruction on means of maintaining health. Also noting the impact of financial well-being on retirement adjustment, they advocated a greater emphasis on financial planning for retirement. They pointed out that many in the baby boom generation are in a precarious position with regard to retirement funds; they also noted that research shows that those who most need this planning—those in lower paying and lower skilled jobs—are also the least likely to plan. Therefore, organizations should be persistent in offering both internal and external resources for this. Taylor and Doverspike also argued that retirement planning should include ensuring that retirees understand the importance of supportive social relationships, because they can buffer the stress of retirement.

Finally, Szinovacz (2003) highlighted the stress that results when retirement does not proceed according to plan because of adverse circumstances. Coping with such circumstances also seems an appropriate topic for retirement planning.

Retirement planning cannot be completely left to the organization. Self-management of retirement will become more important for the same reasons that self-management of career is becoming important (H. L. Sterns & Gray, 1999). Indeed, laws and economic forces have for many already put into self-management one important component of retirement planning—the accumulation and management of retirement funds. A fulfilling retirement will come to depend on individuals planning other parts of their retirement experience as well.

Conclusion

In this chapter and the preceding one, we have made recommendations for organizations that wish to make full use of older workers as part of their workforces. This chapter included the roles of training, performance appraisal, career management, and retirement planning. Although discussed separately, they are actually interrelated; for example, performance appraisal often signals the need for training or career development issues.

Our bias in these chapters is evident: We strongly advocate that organizations begin the process of adapting to an older workforce. This process represents a fundamental change for most organizations, and we recommend that they begin before the demographic crisis. Although business necessity will ultimately force the change, we draw attention as well to the staggering social cost that is being experienced now as older workers are forced from productive and satisfying activity by archaic work structures predicated on decades-old economic arrangements, views of human capabilities, and life expectancies.

There is increasing evidence that work enhances the functioning, well-being, and perhaps even the life span of older persons. For example, Schaie (1994), Schooler et al. (1998), and Warr (1998, 2001) have noted that cognitive function seems to decline when older workers are removed from challenging environments. In addition, House (1998), commenting on his own research, said, "Across the full age range, we observed the greatest physical and psychological well-being in those who are doing as much paid work as they would like to do" (p. 302). Even before the business necessity is felt, we hope that the social necessity will motivate action.

9

A Look Back and
a Look Toward the Future

The world of work continues to change and evolve, promising that the human resource (HR) landscape of tomorrow will be vastly different and ever more challenging. Demographic trends, in particular, require a rethinking of employment and retirement policies to better meet the needs of older workers. Given the centrality that work holds for most individuals, these changing occupational trends and retirement patterns—and changing motivations and capabilities of workers as they age—suggest that the aging workforce will have an important impact on the world of work.

Age discrimination continues to be pervasive in the American workplace. It is beyond question that ageism can play a particularly harmful role in organizations. Older workers face widely held societal stereotypes that are detrimental to morale and productivity. Although adherence to the Age Discrimination in Employment Act (ADEA) is necessary to avoid costly lawsuits, a commitment to the law is insufficient to ensure the sort of changes to the corporate culture that will lead to optimal use of an aging workforce. Management must also be committed to the principle behind the law that each person ought to be judged on individual merit and to be provided with equal opportunity to make the best contribution to the workplace.

Workers in middle and later career and life stages represent a relatively untapped resource in the U.S. workforce. The use of older workers can help organizations meet their growing and changing company objectives in a global economy while providing meaningful work roles for middle-aged and older Americans. To attract sufficient numbers of employees over the next quarter of a century, HR managers will have to include older individuals in the pool of potential employees, and they will have to understand how older workers' needs and motivations differ from those of younger workers. To retain and best utilize the older worker, organizations will need to gain a better understanding of issues surrounding skills and knowledge obsolescence, the need for development of new knowledge and skills, an understanding of the importance of creating new opportunities for employment, and how to motivate and reward different age groups in the workforce.

Changes, Stages, and Opportunities

Aging workers are highly diverse. We begin our work lives with a unique profile of abilities—physical, cognitive, and psychological. As our work lives progress, the nature and trajectory of age-related change vary considerably. In addition, as the nature of work and the nature of the workplace evolve, increased demands for technical and interpersonal skills are placed on workers. H. L. Sterns and Miklos (1995) have suggested that an individual's vocational potential, at any point in his or her career, reflects a unique combination of age-related and non-age-related influences, which they group into normative and nonnormative factors. The normative factors include biological and environmental determinants that bear a strong relationship to chronological age and history-relevant influences that affect most members of a cohort in similar ways. Nonnormative factors include unique career and life changes as well as individual health and stress-inducing events.

Applying their life span development perspective to later work life, H. L. Sterns and Mikos suggested that older workers have the potential for growth and change at anytime in their worklives. In fact, because these factors affect behavioral change during the course of a career, it is important to recognize that individual differences become more pronounced with increasing age. Consequently, the organization's focus should be on a worker's ability and expertise rather than on stereotypic age-related expectations, and its HR policies and procedures should reflect an understanding of both these normative and nonnormative influences on an individual's development and abilities.

It seems quite reasonable, then, that employers should assume that workers of all ages would likely benefit from training programs, opportunities to take on challenging developmental assignments, and interventions aimed at organizational change. Hansson, DeKoekkoek, Neece, and Patterson (1997) have suggested that age-related changes should be viewed from an adaptation perspective, offering older workers numerous opportunities. Older workers, then, should think in terms of continued career aspirations and involvements, and training should focus on that unique potential.

Still, several decades of organizational downsizing and restructuring in the United States have forced workers of all ages to adapt to decreased job, career, and work environment security. Adaptation is difficult in an environment where older workers may be subjected to age stereotyping, age discrimination, and pressure to retire. In such an environment, older workers may become convinced that their skills are becoming obsolete, that training is unavailable, and that much of their organizational value may not be particularly transferable (Hansson et al., 1997).

Indeed, career-stage theorists historically have tended to label late career as a time for "decline and disengagement." Consonant with such views, organizations expect older workers to adjust to their "changing circumstances" by accepting reduced levels of power and new roles based on perceptions of declining competence and motivation and by learning to embrace a life that is less dominated by work. Hall and Mirvis (1995) argued, however, that traditional models of adult and career development do not adequately account for the larger environmental context that plays such an influential role in determining career patterns today. Instead, they underscored the notion that the current work environment is characterized by *change* and *complexity*. Change is both rapid and turbulent; complexity results from more demanding life roles (e.g., employee, spouse, caretaker for children, caretaker for parents) and new technologies. The adaptable employee must have a skill set defined by both depth and variety in order to match the complexities of the work environment. It can also be argued that this increasing need for variety and depth of experience should enhance the perceived value of the older worker, because it takes time to accumulate both. Hall and Mirvis (1995) saw this idea of career flexibility and autonomy as ideal for the older worker because many of the external constraints (e.g., children's education) and internal drives (e.g., advancement) are less likely to dictate behavior. As long as health care and other basic needs are met, the older worker may be freer to pursue more flexible career options than many younger workers.

Career Progression and the Older Worker

Farr, Tesluk, and Klein (1998) suggested that the reality of the current work environment is that organizations can no longer promise steady upward mobility or lifelong employment. Instead, these ever-changing work conditions require employees to be continually adapting to the demands of novel situations and continually learning new skills and acquiring new knowledge. This then leads the authors to suggest that the career of the future will involve periodic cycles of skill learning, mastery, and "reskilling" in order to transition into new positions, jobs, and assignments. Consequently, career growth becomes a function of continuous development and use of new skills and abilities that equip individuals to assume new assignments and positions as needs arise.

Given the present work environment and current knowledge of the needs and capabilities of older workers, Hall and Mirvis (1995) reexamined some traditional models of later career stages. They suggested that the psychological contract between employee and employer has changed in fundamental ways. It is no longer epitomized by the *organizational career*, where people work for one organization until retirement (with that organization valuing seniority and maturity). Instead, any contract between employer and employee is dictated by what they call a *protean career*, a career characterized by variability, adjustment, and change. This new type of career focus allowed the authors to emphasize a more flexible, mobile career course rather than the more traditional notion of linear progression through a series of predictable, discrete career stages. The protean career concept provides a new way of thinking about the relationship between the organization and the employee, with organizations merely providing a context in which individuals can pursue their personal aspirations. A fundamental precept of the new type of psychological contract is that a worker's needs and career concerns change in dynamic ways over the course of a career. One of the keys, therefore, is whether and how workers in midlife can successfully adopt a continual learning and adaptation mode. If the older person is proficient at self-assessment and can engage in a personal "needs analysis," then the chances are much better for successful midcareer transitions and a good match with the new work environment. H. L. Sterns and Miklos (1995) noted that much of the attention on older workers has centered on training rather than longer term career development, and such a perspective offers a rather limited view of the needs and potential contributions of older workers. Instead, they believe that it is important to use a broader perspective that allows identification of deeper developmental needs in ways that promote continuous learning.

Finally, Hall and Mirvis (1995) argued that careers will be increasingly driven by the changing skill demands of the fields in which a person works. Where the life cycle of technologies and products is short, so too will be a worker's personal mastery cycles. People's careers will become increasingly a succession of "mini-learning stages," consisting of exploration–trial–mastery–exit, as they move in and out of product areas, technologies, work groups, organizations, and work environments. Consequently, one set of career stages spanning a lifetime is replaced by a series of many shorter learning cycles. The key component that defines a learning stage will not be chronological age, but career age, where perhaps 5 years in a given specialty may characterize "midlife" for that area. Thus, careers would no longer be measured by the life span of people but by the life span of competencies.

Still, H. L. Sterns and Kaplan (2003) have suggested that older workers may not be as well suited as younger workers to embracing greater career self-management. After all, many older workers initially entered the workforce with a one-career/one-employer ideal, and transitioning from an organization-driven career to a protean career may be a daunting task. Many of the present 50- and 60-year-olds were hired at a time when they could choose among jobs, and they expected that they would have control over how long they worked and when they exited the workforce. Now, many middle-aged and older workers are surprised that the general trend of downsizing—early buyouts and layoffs—has continued, even by many successful companies. This, in combination with recent economic developments, has diminished their investments and led to changes in thinking about retirement plans. Clearly, the decision to continue to work or retire is influenced by many factors.

Thoughts About Retirement

It is important to appreciate the complexity of the retirement decision. Increasingly, retirement transitions are rarely simple or easy but are characterized by multiple exits and reentries into the workforce. Growing numbers of older workers are not simply selecting between continued employment and retirement, but instead are choosing to pursue a variety of options in-between. Certainly, these choices are influenced by the physical and cognitive consequences of aging, the evolving person–environment fit of the employee with the workplace, as well as various social and economic factors. There is an increasing tendency toward "blurred" rather than "crisp" exits from the workforce. As Hansson et al. (1997) have noted, for many older workers retirement involves not so much a line to be crossed as they age but rather a status to be pondered thoughtfully. The removal of a mandatory retirement age for most occupations has increased individual flexibility and responsibility in deciding when and how to exit the workforce. More options are available than ever before to workers and require individuals to manage their careers more proactively (H. L. Sterns & Gray, 1999).

A growing option for older workers is some form of part-time or bridge employment. Weckerle and Schultz (1999) examined factors associated with retirement (continued full-time employment in the present job, bridge employment in the present type of work, or bridge employment in a different type of work) for workers 50 years of age or older who had been in their current job at least 10 years. They found that workers' perceptions of their current and expected financial situation were the most consistent factors that influenced their thoughts and actions. Those who were considering early retirement were more satisfied with their current financial situation, those who were less satisfied with their future financial prospects were considering continued full-time employment, and those whose average financial satisfaction fell between the other two groups were most likely to be considering some form of bridge employment.

The concept of bridge employment complicates the traditional view that older workers simply move from employment to retirement. Traditionally, retirement has meant the "end of work" at the completion of a career or withdrawal from the workforce altogether. More recently, this conceptualization has begun to change. In part, because of the growing popularity of bridge employment, it has become more difficult to distinguish between individuals who are retired and those who are not. Consequently, Feldman (1994) redefined *retirement* to emphasize exit from a position or career path after having spent a considerable length of time in a position, taken by a worker at middle age or beyond to reduce their psychological commitment to work.

It is strikingly clear that older workers want options other than an all-or-nothing retirement or the typical bridge jobs available to older workers. Flexible work alternatives and productive bridge jobs that use the capabilities and experience of older workers are important ways to address this need. Another is phased retirement, an option offered by relatively few organizations (Hansson et al., 1997), one that may prove useful for both older workers and their employers.

Existing retirement policy and philosophy represents a tremendous waste of productive resources and needless trauma to older persons. Within the next 10 years, organizations will begin to feel the labor shortages that will come with the aging workforce. Means that we have discussed to retain older workers—flexible work arrangements, flexible compensation, training and retraining, and career management—will evolve out of necessity. We urge organizations to begin putting these processes in place now.

Retirement rarely occurs for one reason alone. Usually, a number of variables interact to influence the decision to retire, thus suggesting a need for more comprehensive models of the retirement process that examine a larger set of variables and their interactions. With an ever-growing contingent of older workers suggesting they will likely continue to work past traditional retirement age, it becomes all the more important that we increase our efforts to develop a comprehensive understanding of older workers, the nature of their interactions with work and the organizations for which they work, and the process of transitioning to retirement. Organizations must become more knowledgeable and proactive in developing explicit policies regarding their employment of older workers.

The Psychology of Retirement

Healthy adults spend a large portion of their time and energy working. As noted by Forteza and Prieto (1994), these work activities provide considerable structure to their lives, often determining things like schedules and how they distribute their time throughout the day. An individual's repertoire of aptitudes, skills, knowledge, competence, and creativity plays an important role in the behaviors and attitudes he or she displays at work. In addition, a large portion of personal interactions occur in the work setting, and generally some measure of an individual's stature and influence is derived from work. Consequently, decisions pertaining to retirement and its consequences must also be interpreted in light of the meaning that work has for those who continue working and for those who have stopped working.

Friedan (1993) suggested that the transition period from late career to retirement is all too often debilitating for older workers. Because they are too often blocked from participating in the mainstream of work activities after a certain age—at least at levels that would really use the abilities of their age and experience—older workers over time begin to feel less confident about their abilities or less willing to contribute to the organization in meaningful ways.

Even in society, older individuals are often no longer perceived as being active producers and shapers of meaningful substance, but rather as passive dependents on others and on the services that may in fact help to foster greater dependence. From this perspective, Friedan (1993) saw it as not at all surprising that older workers might not want to continue in a rigid, nine-to-five job for an organization that denied them the training that would have allowed them to master new technologies or bypassed them for a promotion in spite of years of experience and expertise. Nevertheless, it is not always possible for older workers to retire from a job or to leave an organization that has treated them unfairly. Workers often do not have the option of retirement without a significant financial sacrifice, and they may not be interested in moving to lower status, low-paying jobs.

Beehr and Bowling (2002) have suggested that an individual's perception of whether his or her retirement is voluntary or involuntary has both physical and psychological ramifications. For example, perceiving retirement as involuntary has been linked to problems with physical and emotional health, depression, and general life and retirement dissatisfaction. In addition, research examining the impact of downsizing demonstrated that psychological well-being and physical health were both adversely affected by the perception of forced retirement. Conversely, when retirement was perceived as voluntary, the result was greater satisfaction with health, finances, activities, life, marriage, and retirement.

Along these same lines, House (1998) noted that at higher socioeconomic levels, self-efficacy tends to decline modestly with age, especially around the period of retirement. Self-efficacy, however, tends to increase with age at lower socioeconomic levels, again most notably in the postretirement years. He suggested that these findings might reflect the different experience and meaning of retirement for people at different socioeconomic levels. For those at higher socioeconomic levels, retirement often results in the loss of a position that had allowed them to acquire esteem, autonomy, and self-direction; at lower socioeconomic levels, retirement often means escaping from a role lacking these positive attributes and experiencing new work opportunities or leisure roles that are more conducive to a sense of self-efficacy.

Szinovacz (2003) proposed the concept of pathways into retirement to convey the notion that retirement decisions reflect long-term and sequential processes. This dynamic view of retirement processes suggests that transitions are imbedded in societal and organizational structures and are tied to people's past and current experiences. Thus, retirement decisions evolve not only from occupational and employment experiences but also from a variety of contextual influences and lifelong experiences in work and nonwork realms. As Szinovacz (2003) noted, one challenge to retirement research is to untangle these dynamics and complexities, including those associated with changing retirement policies and cohort flow.

Public and Private Policy and Retirement

Despite the aging of the U.S. labor force, public and private policies aimed at encouraging older workers to continue their employment are not prevalent. Public policy debate, related to the older worker, has in recent years focused on how extending work life might help alleviate some of the growing public cost of retirement. Those who argued in favor of extending work life beyond age 65 have emphasized legal, demographic, economic, health, and psychological factors as important considerations for permitting greater individual flexibility in choosing to work or retire. Those who argued from a pro-business perspective have tended to suggest that mandatory retirement at age 65 provides a good opportunity for older workers (whose performance levels they assumed may have deteriorated badly) to retire with dignity. They have also suggested that permitting older workers to postpone retirement might "clog" promotion ladders and reduce opportunities for other (younger) employees (Rosen & Jerdee, 1985).

Government efforts at encouraging longer working lives can be found in several pieces of federal legislation. Two specific amendments to the Social Security Act (Social Security Act of 1935, 2004) in 1983 were designed to promote later retirement by (a) increasing the delayed retirement credit and (b) gradually increasing the age of eligibility for full Social Security benefits. Congress took another step to promote longer work lives by repealing the Social Security earnings test in 2000, which had resulted in a loss of benefits for earnings above a certain amount for beneficiaries ages 65 to 69. Rix (2001) pointed out that legislation requiring employer-provided health plans to be the first or primary

insurer of Medicare-eligible workers tends to work against efforts to foster longer work lives. The substantially higher costs of
insuring older workers may discourage organizations from retaining or hiring older workers or may prompt them to offer older
workers only part-time work with fewer benefits. A recent ruling
by the Equal Employment Opportunity Commission has provided
new guidance on this issue and may lessen this burden on employers. The ruling provides a narrow exception from ADEA prohibitions against changing health benefits provided to retirees
once they become eligible for Medicare or comparable state programs (Equal Employment Opportunity Commission, 2004).

Although recent surveys have shown that 80% of the baby
boomers say they want to continue to work in retirement, all survey respondents were strongly opposed to raising the age of eligibility for Social Security benefits (AARP, 1998). Nonetheless,
despite lack of public support, Congress seems likely to seriously
consider further increases in retirement age given the impact that
an increase could have on the solvency of the Social Security system if people worked beyond current retirement ages.

Burtless and Quinn (2002) examined current retirement trends
and policies and concluded that in recent years, many public policies and private institutions designed to promote early retirement
have been revised. Mandatory retirement has been outlawed for
most jobs, Social Security is no longer growing more generous,
and company pension plan coverage is no longer increasing. Social Security and private pensions have adopted a more age-neutral perspective, thus reducing the incentives to retire at a particular age, such as age 62 or age 65. In addition, the scheduled
rise in Social Security's normal retirement age over the next
2 decades should, to some extent, encourage later retirements.

Burtless and Quinn (2002) also suggested that for social and
economic reasons, policymakers may want to encourage people
to work longer. First, they noted that increases in life span mean
that workers retiring in their early 60s will continue to be healthy
and productive individuals for a considerable length of time after retirement. Thus, many older Americans might benefit by staying active in the workforce longer because they derive satisfaction from working and from the social relationships they develop
in the workplace. Second, if people continue to retire in their early

60s, they are at a much greater risk of having insufficient incomes as they grow older. Early retirees give up labor income, receive a reduced monthly benefit from Social Security, and lose the opportunity to contribute to an employer-sponsored pension (if one is offered).

Numerous areas in government policies, programs, and regulations can be changed or enhanced to encourage older people to work. Legislation already in place can be enforced to aid this effort. Although many of the policies discussed here may be described as prowork, the intent is not to advocate work obligations for the elderly; rather, it is to promote public policies that provide incentives and reduce barriers for those who are positively inclined to continue working.

Outliving Retirement Savings

The reality resulting from changing mortality rates and from a shift in types of pension coverage means that baby boomers could be in greater danger of outliving their retirement savings than their parents had been, because baby boomers are more likely to be covered by defined contribution retirement plans. Korczyk (2002) noted that the baby boom generation will be among the first retirees to derive all or most of their pension income from such private retirement plans. In 1977, there were twice as many workers participating in defined benefit plans as there were participating in defined contribution plans. By 1997, that trend had been completely reversed.

From the employees' perspective, the dangers are that defined contribution plans are often optional for the employees, are not designed to replace a specific proportion of preretirement income, and typically do not pay out benefits in annuity form. Consequently, by not participating in the plan, not contributing enough, or investing too conservatively, workers risk not accumulating sufficient retirement income or spending their money too quickly when they do retire.

Korczyk (2002) also pointed out that increased longevity may have a more financially deleterious effect on middle and upper income Americans than on those in lower income groups. Because social security benefits replace a higher proportion of pre-retirement earnings for lower income than for middle and higher income workers, individuals who get the bulk of their retirement income from Social Security will have inflation-protected income that lasts as long as they live. Middle and upper income workers, however, not only tend to live longer but also to depend on employer-sponsored pension plans for a greater share of their retirement income than workers at the lower end of the income scale. Consequently, lower income groups face less financial risk from unexpectedly long retirements than those in the middle and upper income groups do.

A recent AARP (2003) report described a financially secure retirement as being composed of four pillars: Social Security, private pensions and personal savings, earnings, and health insurance. The study also suggested that economic, financial, demographic, and health care trends have combined in recent years to erode the foundation underlying each of the four pillars. In particular, the escalating costs of health care and the cutbacks in employer-sponsored retiree health coverage have made it more difficult for workers to plan for and pay for major medical costs after retirement.

Rix (2001) has suggested that the longer term prospects are good that older workers will be given the opportunity to work longer if they wish. If true, older workers should see an increase in employment opportunities, such as more and better part-time jobs with attractive wages and benefits, job-sharing programs, phased retirement programs, greater use of retiree job banks and rehiring programs, increased use of alternative work schedules, and generous family leave benefits to care for aged relatives. The demographics are certainly in their favor, and Rix contended that history has shown that when employers need workers they will do whatever is necessary to attract them, even if it means taking another look at the very workers they had ignored in the past.

Conclusion

Recent research on careers has focused on how changing organizational contexts (such as downsizing, redefinitions of the psychological contract, increased technology, and globalization) have altered the ways that individuals think about themselves, their careers, and their definitions of career success. As important as these career forces are, Feldman (2002) wisely noted that the aging process itself should not be ignored, because it creates conditions that energize individuals to reconsider and modify their career paths. Thus, although external changes in organizational contexts clearly influence individuals' interests, values, and skills, the maturation process itself stimulates many of the changes in careers we see in individuals over a life span.

Shifts in demographics should prompt a change in the traditional workforce model that endorsed the continual replacement of experienced older workers with a larger number of younger and more educated workers. For the first time, new workers coming into the workforce are likely to be insufficient in numbers and to be no more educated than their predecessors. Employers will be challenged to adopt innovative strategies geared specifically toward the needs of an aging workforce to ensure retention of critical retirement-age employees and the knowledge and expertise that they bring to the workplace.

Faced with a shrinking pool of younger workers to replace those who are retiring, employers must focus on retention of key talent—aging employees with special expertise, key relationships, or difficult to replace skills. In the coming years, employers and older workers will need to work together to design a more fluid retirement model to address the needs of all concerned. In addition, it should not be forgotten that with women becoming an ever-increasing component of the workforce, an understanding of how they might affect retirement models is also important. As Taylor and Doverspike (2003) have suggested, specific predictors of retirement behaviors may interact with gender and thus the very nature of retirement may change.

Robson (2001) has suggested that the tight labor market of the late 1990s provided a glimpse of what is in store for the workplace in the near future. Although the more recent economic slowdown of the early 2000s has depressed the demand for workers, the declining stock market has also depleted the nest eggs that were helping to finance the rapid departures of many older people from the workforce. Together, these trends suggest that the need for advance planning and encouragement of good public policy is still pressing.

Although discussion continues about needed changes in policies to guarantee the viability of old-age security, policy changes can succeed only if they are complemented by changes in other domains. Viewed from a strategic HR management perspective, scarcer labor will simply underscore the need for organizational policies and practices that already make good business sense: that is, attracting and retaining people with the optimal combination of knowledge, skills, and abilities.

The ability of organizations to incorporate innovative hiring strategies, flexible work schedules, training, imaginative compensation and business structures, and new workplace technologies will all contribute to retaining key talent. Employers who do not adapt to a changing workforce will lose their edge in recruiting and find workers (young and old) leaving for competitors. Employers and governments that respond early and energetically to this emerging workforce challenge will gain a key competitive advantage.

Regardless of the changes organizations make in the structure and functioning of the workplace of the future, almost certainly the older worker will play a crucial role. For their part, older workers will need to improve their work skills through education and training. The likely result of such commitment might be lifelong retraining so as to combat skill obsolescence (D. A. Peterson & Wendt, 1995). In turn, organizations need to make it worthwhile for older employees to continue to be productive and to gain satisfaction from their work activities so that all of those concerned achieve a positive outcome (Shea, 1991).

Because of the importance of financial security for older workers, pension benefits are likely to play a primary role when these workers are faced with the choice of either retiring or adapting to a changing work environment. Older workers with pensions must carefully compare the costs and benefits of remaining as opposed to retiring. For some workers, the availability of adequate pension benefits will make retirement an attractive option, and if the retirement option is perceived to be more lucrative than remaining on the job, the probability that an older worker will choose to remain and adapt is considerably reduced. For others, the lack of adequate pension benefits may increase the anxiety brought about by workplace changes (Yeatts, Folts, & Knapp, 2000).

Each of us is an aging worker, and each of us has a stake in how the aging workforce changes the structure of jobs, work incentives, and retirement (Mitchell, 1993). As the baby boomers move rapidly toward retirement age, concepts such as "productive aging" and "active aging" receive more frequent mention in the popular press. Older adults want to continue to stay involved in work life in meaningful roles. They wish to use their potential, contribute to their families and communities, and preserve their health and well-being. Certainly, there is a growing realization of the integral role these workers will play in the labor force of the future. In addition, the decline in traditional career trajectories, technological advancements that encourage work from home (among other changes), as well as evolving policies encouraging greater use of older workers render boundaries between work and other life spheres less definite and more variable.

In this book we have tried to present and discuss the challenges and opportunities facing organizations as their workforce ages. As employees age, they want to be paid and rewarded in different ways, including coverage for costly health care. These changing expectations must be recognized and addressed by organizations and their employees over the next few decades. Government and private retirement programs, particularly pension plans and Social Security, must also be prepared to meet the new demands.

Healthy adults spend a major portion of their time and energy engaged in work activities. Consequently, it makes sense for organizational psychologists to invest time and energy in examining more closely the many issues arising from an aging workforce and in understanding more clearly the capabilities, motivations, interests, and expectations of this ever-increasing proportion of the labor force. Indeed, many challenges remain for the future. We need to gain a better understanding of how aging interacts with skills, abilities, interests, motivations, incentives, retirement and pension policies, HR policies, and many other important issues. Currently, our knowledge of these processes comes from a diverse set of research disciplines. Much remains to be learned about aging workers; the forces that influence their decisions; and how their knowledge, skills, and experience can be harnessed for the benefit of organizations and society. The coming decades promise to be an extremely dynamic and challenging period for organizations and their aging workforce.

References

AARP. (1998, June). *Boomers look toward retirement*. Washington, DC: Author.

AARP. (1999). *Easing the transition: Phased and partial retirement programs*. Washington, DC: Author.

AARP. (2001). *Beyond 50: A report to the nation on economic security*. Washington, DC: Author.

AARP. (2002). *Flexible ways of working*. Retrieved September 21, 2003, from http://www.aarp.org/careers-tools/articles-a2002-12-12-flexwork.html

AARP. (2003). *Staying ahead of the curve 2003: The AARP working in retirement study*. Washington, DC: AARP, Knowledge Management.

AARP Work Link Team Program Development and Services. (2000, January). *American business and older employees: A summary of findings*. Washington, DC: AARP Research Center.

Abraham, J. D., & Hansson, R. O. (1995). Successful aging at work: An applied study of selection, optimization, and compensation through impression management. *Journal of Gerontology: Psychological Sciences, 50,* 94–103.

Adams v. Florida Power, 535 U.S. 228 (2002).

Age Discrimination in Employment Act of 1967, 29 U.S.C. § 621 *et seq.* (2004).

Applebaum, E., & Gregory, J. (1990). Flexible employment: Union perspectives. In P. B. Doeringer (Ed.), *Bridges to retirement: Older workers in a changing labor market* (pp. 130–145). Ithaca, NY: ILR Press.

Arbuckle, T. Y., Gold, D., & Andres, D. (1986). Cognitive functioning of older people in relation to social and personality variables. *Psychology and Aging, 1,* 55–62.

Arkes, H., & Blumer, C. (1985). The psychology of sunk cost. *Organisational Behaviour and Human Decision Processes, 35,* 124–140.

Ashbaugh, D. L., & Fay, C. H. (1987). The threshold for aging in the workplace. *Research on Aging, 9,* 417–427.

Automaker is set to pay $10.5 million in suit. (2001, December 19). *New York Times,* p. C4.

Avolio, B. J., & Waldman, D. A. (1994). Variations in cognitive, perceptual, and psychomotor abilities across the working life span: Examining the effects of race, sex, experience, education, and occupational type. *Psychology and Aging, 9,* 430–442.

Avolio, B. J., Waldman, D. A., & McDaniel, M. A. (1990). Age and work performance in nonmanagerial jobs: The effects of experience and occupation type. *Academy of Management Journal, 32,* 407–422.

Baltes, P. B., & Baltes, M. M. (1990a). Psychological perspectives on successful aging: The model of selective optimization with compensation. In P. B.

Baltes & M. M. Baltes (Eds.), *Successful aging: Perspectives from the behavioral sciences* (pp. 1–34). Cambridge, England: Cambridge University Press.

Baltes, P. B., & Baltes, M. M. (Eds.). (1990b). *Successful aging: Perspectives from the behavioral sciences*. Cambridge, England: Cambridge University Press.

Baltes, P., Dittman-Kohli, F., & Kliegl, R. (1986). Reserve capacity of the elderly in aging-sensitive tests of fluid intelligence: Replication and extension. *Psychology and Aging, 1,* 172–177.

Barnes, D. E., Yaffe, K., Satariano, W. A., & Tager, I. B. (2003). A longitudinal study of cardio-respiratory fitness and cognitive function in healthy older adults. *Journal of the American Geriatrics Society, 51,* 459–465.

Barrett, G. V., & Kernan, M. C. (1987). Performance appraisal and terminations: A review of court decisions since Brito v. Zia with implications for personnel practices. *Personnel Psychology, 40,* 489–503.

Barrick, M. R., Mount, M. K., & Judge, T. A. (2001). Personality and performance at the beginning of the new millennium: What do we know and where do we go next? *International Journal of Selection and Assessment, 9,* 9–30.

Barringer, M. W., & Mitchell, O. S. (1993). Health insurance choice and the older worker. In O. S. Mitchell (Ed.), *As the workforce ages: Costs, benefits, and policy challenges* (pp. 125–146). Ithaca, NY: ILR Press.

Barth, M. C., McNaught, W., & Rizzi, P. (1995). Older Americans as workers. In S. A. Bass (Ed.), *Older and active: How Americans over 55 are contributing to society* (pp. 35–70). New Haven, CT: Yale University Press.

Bass, S. A., Quinn, J. F., & Burkhauser, R. V. (1995). Toward pro-work policies and programs for older Americans. In S. A. Bass (Ed.), *Older and active: How Americans over 55 are contributing to society* (pp. 263–294). New Haven, CT: Yale University Press.

Beehr, T. A., & Adams, G. A. (2003). Introduction and overview of current research and thinking on retirement. In G. A. Adams & T. A. Beehr (Eds.), *Retirement: Reasons, processes, and results* (pp. 1–5). New York: Springer Publishing Company.

Beehr, T. A., & Bowling, N. A. (2002). Career issues facing older workers. In D. Feldman (Ed.), *Work careers: A developmental perspective* (pp. 214–241). San Francisco: Jossey-Bass.

Belous, R. S. (1990). Flexible employment: The employer's point of view. In P. B. Doeringer (Ed.), *Bridges to retirement: Older workers in a changing labor market* (pp. 111–128). Ithaca, NY: ILR Press.

Birdi, K. M., Warr, P. B., & Oswald, A. J. (1995). Age differences in three components of employee well-being. *Applied Psychology: An International Review, 44,* 345–373.

Block, J. (1971). *Lives through time*. Berkeley, CA: Bancroft Books.

Borman, W. C. (1991). Job behavior, performance, and effectiveness. In M. D. Dunnette & L. M. Hough (Eds.), *Handbook of industrial and organizational psychology* (pp. 271–326). Palo Alto, CA: Consulting Psychologists Press.

Borman, W. C., & Motowidlo, S. M. (1993). Expanding the criterion domain to include elements of contextual performance. In N. Schmitt & W. C. Borman (Eds.), *Personnel selection* (pp. 71–98). San Francisco: Jossey-Bass.

Borman, W. C., Penner, L. A., Allen, T. D., & Motowidlo, S. J. (2001). Personality predictors of citizenship performance. *International Journal of Selection and Assessment, 9,* 52–69.

Bosma, H., van Boxtel, M. P. J., Ponds, R. W. H. M., Houx, P. S. H., & Jolles, J. (2003). Education and age-related cognitive decline: The contribution of mental workload. *Educational Gerontology, 29,* 165–173.

Bosma, H., van Boxtel, M. P. J., Ponds, R. W. H. M., Jelicic, M., Houx, P. S. H., Metsemakers, J., & Jolles, J. (2002). Engaged lifestyle and cognitive function in middle and old-aged, non-demented persons: A reciprocal association? *Journal for the German Society of Gerontology and Geriatrics, 35,* 575–581.

Bovbjerg, B., Jeszeck, C., & Petersen, J. (2001, November). *Older workers: Demographic trends pose challenges for employers and workers.* Report to the ranking minority member, Subcommittee on Employer–Employee Relations, Committee on Education and the Workforce, House of Representatives (GAO Report No. GAO-02-85). Washington, DC: General Accounting Office.

Brandstädter, J., & Rothermund, K. (1994). Self-percepts of control in middle and later adulthood: Buffering losses by rescaling goals. *Psychology and Aging, 9,* 265–273.

Brandstädter, J., Wentura, D., & Rothermund, K. (1999). Intentional self-development through adulthood and later life: Tenacious pursuit and flexible adjustment of goals. In J. Brandstädter & R. M. Lerner (Eds.), *Action and self-development: Theory and research through the life span* (pp. 373–400). Thousand Oaks, CA: Sage Publications.

Bridges, W. (1994, September 19). The end of the job. *Fortune, 130*(6), 62–74.

Brown, G. (1992). Spring wind. On *Dream café* [record]. St. Paul, MN: Red House Records.

Bryk, A. S., & Raudenbush, S.W. (1987). Application of hierarchical linear models to assessing change. *Psychological Bulletin, 101,* 147–158.

Burkhauser, R. V., & Quinn, J. F. (1983). Is mandatory retirement overrated? Evidence from the 1970s. *Journal of Human Resources, 18,* 337–358.

Burtless, G. (1993). The fiscal challenge of an aging population. In O. Mitchell (Ed.), *As the workforce ages: Costs, benefits, and policy challenges* (pp. 225–252). Ithaca, NY: ILR Press.

Burtless, G., & Quinn, J. F. (2001). Retirement trends and policies to encourage work among older Americans. In P. P. Budetti, R. V. Burkhauser, J. M. Gregory, & H. A. Hunt (Eds.), *Ensuring health and income security for an aging workforce* (pp. 375–415). Kalamazoo, MI: W. E. Upjohn Institute for Employment Research.

Burtless, G., & Quinn, J. F. (2002). *Is working longer the answer for an aging workforce?* Boston: Boston College Center for Retirement Research.

Canaff, A. L. (1997). Later life career planning: A new challenge for counselors. *Journal of Employment Counseling, 34*, 85–94.

Capowski, G. (1994). Ageism: The new diversity issue. *Management Review, 83*, 10–15.

Chan, S., & Stevens, A. H. (2001). Job loss and employment patterns of older workers. *Journal of Labor Economics, 19*, 484–522.

Christensen, K. (1990). Bridges over troubled water: How older workers view the labor market. In P. B. Doeringer (Ed.), *Bridges to retirement: Older workers in a changing labor market* (pp. 175–207). Ithaca, NY: ILR Press.

Civil Rights Act of 1964, Title VII, 42 U.S.C. § 2000e *et seq.* (2003).

Clark, A. E., & Oswald, A. J. (1996). Satisfaction and comparison income. *Journal of Public Economics, 61*, 359–381.

Cleveland, J. N., Festa, R. M., & Montgomery, L. (1988). Applicant pool composition and job perceptions: Impact on decisions regarding an older applicant. *Journal of Vocational Behavior, 32*, 112–125.

Cleveland, J. N., & Hollman, G. (1990). The effects of the age-type of tasks and incumbent age composition on job perceptions. *Journal of Vocational Behavior, 36*, 181–194.

Cleveland, J. N., & Shore, L. M. (1992). Self- and supervisory perspectives on age and work attitudes and performance. *Journal of Applied Psychology, 77*, 469–484.

Cohen, A. (2003, March 2). Too old to work? *New York Times*, p. 54.

Copeland, C. (2004, October). *Employment-based retirement plan participation: Geographic differences and trends* (EBRI Issue Brief No. 274). Washington, DC: Employee Benefit Research Institute.

Costa, P. T., Jr., & McCrae, R. R. (1980). Still stable after all these years: Personality as a key to some issues in adulthood and old age. In P. B. Baltes & O. G. Brim Jr. (Eds.), *Life span development and behavior* (Vol. 3, pp. 65–102). New York: Academic Press.

Costa P. T., Jr., & McCrae, R. R. (1985). *The NEO Personality Inventory manual.* Odessa, FL: Psychological Assessment Resources.

Czaja, S. J. (1996). Aging and the acquisition of computer skills. In W. A. Rogers & A. D. Fisk (Eds.), *Aging and skilled performance: Advances in theory and applications* (pp. 201–220). Mahwah, NJ: Erlbaum.

Czaja, S. J. (2001). Technological change and the older worker. In J. E. Birren & K. W. Schaie (Eds.), *Handbook of the psychology of aging* (pp. 547–568). San Diego, CA: Academic Press.

Czaja, S. J., & Moen, P. (2004). Technology and employment. In R. Pew & S. Van Hemel (Eds.), *Technology for adaptive aging: Report and papers* (pp. 150–178). Washington, DC: National Academies Press.

Czaja, S. J., & Sharit, J. (1993). Age differences in the performance of computer-based work. *Psychology and Aging, 8*, 59–67.

Czaja, S. J., & Sharit, J. (1998). Ability–performance relationships as a function of age and task experience for a data entry task. *Journal of Experimental Psychology: Applied, 4*, 332–351.

Deary, I. J., Whalley, L. J, & Starr, J. M. (2003). IQ at age 11 and longevity: Results from a follow-up of the Scottish Mental Survey 1932. In C. Finch, J. M. Robine, & Y. Christen (Eds.), *Brain and longevity: Perspectives in longevity* (pp. 153–164). Berlin: Springer-Verlag.

Deary, I. J., Whiteman, M. C., Starr, J. M., Whalley, L. J, & Fox, H. (2004). The impact of childhood intelligence on later life: Following up the Scottish Mental Surveys of 1932 and 1947. *Journal of Personality and Social Psychology, 86,* 130–147.

Dennis, H. (Ed.). (1988a). *Fourteen steps in managing an aging work force.* Lexington, MA: Lexington Books.

Dennis, H. (1988b). Management training. In H. Dennis (Ed.), *Fourteen steps in managing an aging work force* (pp. 141–154). Lexington, MA: Lexington Books.

Dennis, H. (1988c). Retirement planning. In H. Dennis (Ed.), *Fourteen steps in managing an aging work force* (pp. 215–229). Lexington, MA: Lexington Books.

DeViney, S., & O'Rand, A. M. (1988). Gender cohort succession and retirement among older men and women, 1951–1984. *Sociological Quarterly, 29,* 525–540.

Diehl, M., Coyle, N., & Labouvie-Vief, G. (1996). Age and sex differences in strategies of coping and defense across the life span. *Psychology and Aging, 11,* 127–139.

Doering, M., Rhodes, S. R., & Schuster, M. (1983). *The aging worker: Research and recommendations.* Beverly Hills, CA: Sage Publications.

Doeringer, P. B. (1990). Economic security, labor market flexibility, and bridges to retirement. In P. B. Doeringer (Ed.), *Bridges to retirement: Older workers in a changing labor market* (pp. 3–19). Ithaca, NY: ILR Press.

Doeringer, P. B., & Terkla, D. G. (1990). Business necessity, bridge jobs, and the nonbureaucratic firm. In P. B. Doeringer (Ed.), *Bridges to retirement: Older workers in a changing labor market* (pp. 146–171). Ithaca, NY: ILR Press.

Dohm, A. (2000). Gauging the labor force effects of retiring baby-boomers. *Monthly Labor Review, 123,* 17–25.

Dubin, S. S. (1990). Maintaining competence through updating. In S. L. Willis & S. S. Dubin (Eds.), *Maintaining professional competence: Approaches to career enhancement, vitality, and success throughout a work life* (pp. 9–43). San Francisco: Jossey-Bass.

Duka, W., & Nicholson, T. (2002, December). Retirees rocking old roles. *AARP Bulletin Online.* Retrieved February 5, 2003, from www.aarp.org/bulletin/yourlife/articles/a2003-06-26-retireesrocking.html

Ekerdt, D. J. (1998). Workplace norms for the timing of retirement. In K. W. Schaie & C. Schooler (Eds.), *Impact of work on older adults* (pp. 101–130). New York: Springer Publishing Company.

Ellison, R., Melville, D., & Gutman, R. (1996). British labour force projections: 1996–2006. *Labour Market Trends, 104,* 197–213.

Equal Employment Opportunity Commission. (2004, March 8). *EEOC issues fiscal year 2003 enforcement data*. Retrieved October 30, 2004, from http://eeoc.gov/press/3-08-04.html

Erikson, E. (1959). Identity and the life cycle. *Psychological Issues, 1*, 1–171.

Faley, R. H., Kleiman, L. S., & Lengnick-Hall, M. L. (1984). Age discrimination and personnel psychology: A review and synthesis of the legal literature with implications for future research. *Personnel Psychology, 37*, 327–350.

Farr, J. L., & Middlebrooks, C. L. (1990). Enhancing motivation to participate in professional development. In S. L. Willis & S. S. Dubin (Eds.), *Maintaining professional competence: Approaches to career enhancement, vitality, and success throughout a work life* (pp. 195–213). San Francisco: Jossey-Bass.

Farr, J. L., & Ringseis, E. L (2002). The older worker in organizational context: Beyond the individual. In C. L. Cooper & I. T. Robertson (Eds.), *International review of industrial and organizational psychology* (Vol. 17, pp. 31–76). Chichester, England: John Wiley.

Farr, J. L., Tesluk, P. E., & Klein, S. R. (1998). Organizational structure of the workplace and the older worker. In K. Schaie & C. Schooler (Eds.), *Impact of work on older adults* (pp. 143–185). New York: Springer Publishing Company.

Feldman, D. C. (1994). The decision to retire early: A review and conceptualization. *Academy of Management Review, 19*, 285–311.

Feldman, D. (Ed.). (2002). Stability in the midst of change. In D. Feldman (Ed.), *Work careers: A developmental perspective* (pp. 3–26). San Francisco: Jossey-Bass.

Finkel, D., Reynolds, C. A., McArdle, J. J., Gatz, M., & Pedersen, N. L. (2003). Latent growth curve analyses of accelerating decline in cognitive abilities in adulthood. *Developmental Psychology, 39*, 535–550.

Finkelstein, L. M., Burke, M. J., & Raju, N. S. (1995). Age discrimination in simulated employment contexts: An integrative analysis. *Journal of Applied Psychology, 80*, 652–663.

Fisk, A. D., & Rogers, W. A. (2000). Influence of training and experience on skill acquisition and maintenance in older adults. *Journal of Aging and Physical Activity, 8*, 373–378.

Fleishman, E. A., Costanza, D. P., & Marshall-Mies, J. (1999). Abilities. In N. G. Peterson, M. D. Mumford, W. C. Borman, P. R. Jeanneret, & E. A. Fleishman (Eds.), *An occupational analysis system for the 21st century: The development of O*NET* (pp. 175–195). Washington, DC: American Psychological Association.

Forteza, J. A., & Prieto, J. M. (1994). Aging and work behavior. In H. Triandis, M. Dunnette, & L. Hough (Eds.), *Handbook of industrial and organizational psychology* (2nd ed., Vol. 4, pp. 447–483). Palo Alto, CA: Consulting Psychologists Press.

Freund, A. M., & Baltes, P. B. (1998). Selection, optimization, and compensation as strategies of life management: Correlations with subjective indicators of successful aging. *Psychology and Aging, 13*, 531–543.

Friedan, B. (1993). *The fountain of age*. New York: Simon & Schuster.

Fullerton, H. N., & Toossi, M. (2001). Labor force projections to 2010: Steady growth and changing composition. *Monthly Labor Review, 124,* 21–38.

Fyock, C. D. (1990). *America's work force is coming of age: What every business needs to know to recruit, train, manage, and retain an aging work force.* New York: Lexington Books.

Gilbert, G. R., Collins, R. W., & Valenzi, E. (1993). Relationship of age and job performance: From the eye of the supervisor. *Journal of Employee Assistance Research, 2,* 36–46.

Goldberg, B. (2000). *Age works: What corporate America must do to survive the graying of the workforce.* New York: Free Press.

Goldberg, L. R. (1990). An alternative "description of personality": The Big Five factor structure. *Journal of Personality and Social Psychology, 59,* 1216–1229.

Goldberg, L. R. (1993). The structure of phenotypic personality traits. *American Psychologist, 48,* 26–34.

Gordon, R. A., & Arvey, R. D. (1986). Perceived and actual ages of workers. *Journal of Vocational Behavior, 28,* 21–28.

Gordon, R. A., Arvey, R. D., Hodges, T. L., Sowanda, K. M., & King, C. M. (2000, May). *The issue of generalizability in age discrimination research: A meta-analytic investigation.* Paper presented at the annual conference of the Midwestern Psychological Association, Chicago.

Gough, H. G. (1996). *CPI manual* (3rd ed.). Palo Alto, CA: Consulting Psychologists Press.

Greller, M. M., & Stroh, L. K. (1995). Careers in midlife and beyond: A fallow field in need of sustenance. *Journal of Vocational Behavior, 47,* 232–247.

Greller, M. M., & Stroh, L. K. (2003). Extending work lives: Are current approaches tools or talismans? In G. A. Adams & T. A. Beehr (Eds.), *Retirement: Reasons, processes, and results* (pp. 115–135). New York: Springer Publishing Company.

Gribbin, K., Schaie, K. W., & Parham, I. A. (1980). Complexity of life style and maintenance of intellectual abilities. *Journal of Social Issues, 36,* 47–61.

Gruber, A. L., & Schaie, K. W. (1986, November). *Longitudinal-sequential studies of marital assortativity.* Paper presented at the annual meeting of the Gerontological Society of America, Chicago.

Haan, N., Milsap, R., & Hartka, E. (1986). As time goes by: Change and stability in personality over 50 years. *Psychology and Aging, 1,* 220–232.

Hale, N. (1990). *The older worker: Effective strategies for management and human resource development.* San Francisco: Jossey-Bass.

Hall, D. T., & Mirvis, P. H. (1995). The new career contract: Developing the whole person at midlife and beyond. *Journal of Vocational Psychology, 47,* 269–289.

Hansson, R. O., DeKoekkoek, P. D., Neece, W. M., & Patterson, D. W. (1997). Successful aging at work: Annual review, 1992–1996: The older worker and transitions to retirement. *Journal of Vocational Behavior, 51,* 202–233.

Harlow, R. E., & Cantor, N. (1996). Still participating after all these years: A study of life task participation in later life. *Journal of Personality and Social Psychology, 71,* 1235–1249.

Hassell, B. L., & Perrewe, P. L. (1993). An examination of the relationship between older workers' perceptions of age discrimination and employee psychological states. *Journal of Management Issues, 5*, 109–120.

Hayward, M. D., Grady, W. R., Hardy, M. A., & Sommers, D. (1989). Occupational influences on retirement, disability, and death. *Demography, 26*, 393–409.

Hayward, M. D., Hardy, M. A., & Grady, W. R. (1989). Labor force withdrawal patterns among a cohort of older men in the United States. *Social Science Quarterly, 70*, 425–448.

Hazen Paper Co. v. Biggins, 507 U.S. 604 (1993).

Hecker, D. E. (2001). Occupational employment projections to 2010. *Monthly Labor Review, 124*, 57–84.

Heckhausen, J., & Schultz, R. (1999). Selectivity in life-span development: Biological and societal canalizations and individuals' developmental goals. In J. Brandstädter & R. M. Lerner (Eds.), *Action and self-development: Theory and research through the life span* (pp. 67–103). Thousand Oaks, CA: Sage Publications.

Helson, R., Jones, C., & Kwan, V. S. Y. (2002). Personality change in adulthood: Hierarchical linear modeling analyses of two longitudinal samples. *Journal of Personality and Social Psychology, 83*, 752–766.

Hertzog, C., Schaie, K. W., & Gribbin, K. (1978). Cardiovascular disease and changes in intellectual functioning from middle to old age. *Journal of Gerontology, 33*, 872–883.

House, J. S. (1998). Commentary: Age, work, and well-being: Toward a broader view. In K. W. Schaie & C. Schooler (Eds.), *Impact of work on older adults* (pp. 297–303). New York: Springer Publishing Company.

Howard, A. (1998). Commentary: New careers and older workers. In K. W. Schaie & C. Schooler (Eds.), *Impact of work on older adults* (pp. 235–245). New York: Springer Publishing Company.

Hoyer, W. J. (1998). Commentary: The older individual in a rapidly changing work context: Developmental and cognitive issues. In K. W. Schaie & C. Schooler (Eds.), *Impact of work on older adults* (pp. 28–44). New York: Springer Publishing Company.

Hummert, M. L. (1999). A social cognitive perspective on age stereotypes. In T. M. Hess & F. Blanchard-Fields (Eds.), *Social cognition and aging* (pp. 175–196). San Diego, CA: Academic Press.

Hunter, J. E. (1980). *Validity generalization for 12,000 jobs: An application of synethetic and validity generalization to the General Aptitude Test Battery (GATB)*. Washington, DC: U.S. Department of Labor, Employment Service.

Inkeles, A., & Levinson, D. J. (1963). The personal system and the sociocultural system in large-scale organizations. *Sociometry, 26*, 217–229.

Job Training Partnership Act of 1982, 29 U.S.C. § 1501 *et seq.* (2004).

Johnson, D. F., & White, C. B. (1980). Effects of training on computerized test performance in the elderly. *Journal of Applied Psychology, 65*, 357–358.

Jolles, J., van Boxtel, M. P. J., Ponds, R. W. H. M., Metsemakers, J. F. M., & Houx, P. J. (1998). The Maastricht aging study (MAAS): The longitudinal perspective of cognitive aging. *Tijdschrift voor Gerontologie en Geriatrie, 29,*120–129.

Jones, C. J., & Meredith, W. (1996). Patterns of personality change across the life span. *Psychology and Aging, 11,* 57–65.

Kacmar, K. M., & Ferris, G. R. (1989). Theoretical and methodological considerations in the age–job satisfaction relationship. *Journal of Applied Psychology, 74,* 201–207.

Kaufman, H. G. (1990). Management techniques for maintaining a competent professional work force. In S. L. Willis & S. S. Dubin (Eds.), *Maintaining professional competence: Approaches to career enhancement, vitality, and success throughout a work life* (pp. 249–261). San Francisco: Jossey-Bass.

Kimel v. Florida Board of Regents, 528 U.S. 62 (2000).

Kling, K. C., Seltzer, M. M., & Ryff, C. D. (1997). Adaptive changes in the self-concept during a life transition. *Personality and Social Psychology Bulletin, 23,* 989–998.

Knowles, M. S. (1987). Adult learning. In R. L. Craig (Ed.), *Training and development handbook* (3rd ed., pp. 168–179). New York: McGraw-Hill.

Kohn, M. L., & Schooler, C. (1983). *Work and personality: An inquiry into the impact of social stratification.* Norwood, NJ: Ablex.

Korczyk, S. M. (2002, December). *Back to which future: The U.S. aging crisis revisited* (Report No. 2002-18). Washington, DC: AARP Public Policy Institute.

Kouzes, J., & Posner, B. (1987). *The leadership challenge.* New York: Jossey-Bass.

Kubeck, J. E., Delp, N. D., Haslett, T. K., & McDaniel, M. A. (1996). Does job-related training performance decline with age? *Psychology and Aging, 11,* 92–107.

LaRocco, J. M., House, J. S., & French, J. R. P., Jr. (1980). Social support, occupational stress, and health. *Journal of Health and Social Behavior, 21,* 202–218.

Lawrence, B. S. (1987). An organizational theory of age effects. *Research in the Sociology of Organizations, 5,* 37–71.

Lawrence, B. S. (1988). New wrinkles in the theory of age demography norms and performance ratings. *Academy of Management Journal, 31,* 309–337.

Lawrence, B. S. (1996). Interest and indifference: The role of age in the organizational sciences. In G. R. Ferris (Ed.), *Research in personnel and human resources management* (pp. 1–59). Greenwich, CT: JAI Press.

Levine, M. L. (1988). Age discrimination: The law and its underlying policy. In H. Dennis (Ed.), *Fourteen steps in managing an aging work force* (pp. 25–35). Lexington, MA: Lexington Books.

Levine, P. B. (1993). Examining labor force projections for the twenty-first century. In O. S. Mitchell (Ed.), *As the workforce ages* (pp. 38–56). Ithaca, NY: IRL Press.

Liebig, P. S. (1988). The work force of tomorrow: Its challenge to management. In H. Dennis (Ed.), *Fourteen steps in managing an aging work force* (pp. 3–21). Lexington, MA: Lexington Books.

Malatest, R. A. (2003, February). *The aging workforce and human resources development implications for sector councils.* Ottawa, Ontario, Canada: Malatest & Associates.

Mandatory retirement and chronological age in public safety workers: Testimony before the United States Senate Committee on Labor and Human Resources, 104th Cong., 2 (1996) (testimony of F. J. Landy).

Marshall, V. W. (1998). Commentary: The older worker and organizational restructuring: Beyond systems theory. In K. W. Schaie & C. Schooler (Eds.), *Impact of work on older adults* (pp. 195–206). New York: Springer Publishing Company.

Masunaga, H., & Horn, J. L. (2001). Expertise and age-related changes in components of intelligence. *Psychology and Aging, 16*, 293–311.

Maurer, T. J. (2001). Career-relevant learning and development, worker age, and beliefs about self-efficacy for development. *Journal of Management, 27*, 123–140.

Maurer, T. J., Wrenn, K. A., & Weiss, E. M. (2003). Toward understanding and managing stereotypical beliefs about older workers' ability and desire for learning and development. In J. J. Martocchio & G. R. Ferris (Eds.), *Research in personnel and human resources management* (Vol. 22, pp. 253–285). Stamford, CT: JAI Press.

McAdams, D. P., & de St. Aubin, E. (1998). *Generativity and adult development: How and why we care for the next generation*. Washington, DC: American Psychological Association.

McArdle, J. J., Ferrer-Caja, E., Hamagami, F., & Woodcock, R. W. (2002). Comparative longitudinal structural analyses of the growth and decline of multiple intellectual abilities over the life span. *Developmental Psychology, 38*, 115–142.

McCann, R., & Giles, H. (2002). Ageism in the workplace: A communication perspective. In T. D. Nelson (Ed.), *Ageism: Stereotyping and prejudice against older persons* (pp. 163–199). Cambridge, MA: MIT Press.

McCrae, R. R., Costa, P. T., Jr., de Lima, M. P., Simões, A., Ostendorf, F., Angleitner, A., et al. (1999). Age differences in personality across the adult lifespan: Parallels in five cultures. *Developmental Psychology, 35*, 466–477.

McCrae, R. R., Costa, P. T., Jr., Ostendorf, F., Angleitner, A., Hrebickova, M., Avia, M. D., et al. (2000). Nature over nurture: Temperament, personality, and life span development. *Journal of Personality and Social Psychology, 78*, 173–186.

McDonald, R. B. (1988). The physiological aspects of aging. In H. Dennis (Ed.), *Fourteen steps in managing an aging work force* (pp. 39–51). Lexington, MA: Lexington Books.

McEvoy, G. M., & Cascio, W. F. (1989). Cumulative evidence of the relationship between employee age and job performance. *Journal of Applied Psychology, 74*, 11–17.

McGue, M., Bouchard, T. J., Jr., Iacono, W. G., & Lykken, D. T. (1993). Behavioral genetics of cognitive ability: A life-span perspective. In R. Plomin & G. E. McClearn (Eds.), *Nature, nurture, and psychology* (pp. 59–76). Washington, DC: American Psychological Association.

Menchin, R. S. (2000). *New work opportunities for older Americans*. New York: iUniverse.com, Inc.

Meredith, W., & Tisak, J. (1990). Latent curve analysis. *Psychometrika, 55,* 107–122.

Miller, C. S., Kaspin, J. A., & Schuster, M. H. (1990). The impact of performance appraisal methods on age discrimination in employment act cases. *Personnel Psychology, 43,* 555–578.

Miller, D. B. (1990). Organizational, environmental, and work design strategies that foster competence. In S. L. Willis & S. S. Dubin (Eds.), *Maintaining professional competence: Approaches to career enhancement, vitality, and success throughout a work life* (pp. 214–232). San Francisco: Jossey-Bass.

Miller, D. M., Cox, S., Gieson, M., Bean, C., Adams-Price, C., Sanderson, P., & Topping, J. S. (1993). Further development and validation of an age-based equal opportunity measure for organizations: An operational definition of ecological dissonance. *Psychology: A Journal of Human Behavior, 30,* 32–37.

Mitchell, O. S. (1993). As the workforce ages. In O. S. Mitchell (Ed.), *As the workforce ages: Costs, benefits, and policy challenges* (pp. 3–15). Ithaca, NY: ILR Press.

Mondy, R., Sharplin, A., & Flippo, E. B. (1988). *Management: Concepts and practices.* Boston: Allyn & Bacon.

Montenegro, X., Fisher, L., & Remez, S. (2002, September). *Staying ahead of the curve: The AARP work and career study—A national survey conducted for AARP by RogerASW.* Washington, DC: AARP Knowledge Management.

Morris, M. G., & Venkatesh, V. (2000). Age differences in technology adoption decisions: Implications for a changing work force. *Personnel Psychology, 53,* 375–403.

Morrow, D., Leirer, V., Altiteri, P., & Fitzsimmons, C. (1994). When expertise reduces age differences in performance. *Psychology and Aging, 9,* 134–148.

Moss, H. A., & Susman, E. J. (1980). Constancy and change in personality development. In O. G. Brim & J. Kagan (Eds.), *Constancy and change in human development* (pp. 530–595). Cambridge, MA: Harvard University Press.

Muller, C., & Knapp, K. (2003, May). *Occupations in an aging society: Worker abilities and worker interests.* Paper presented at the International Research Conference on Social Security, Antwerp, Belgium.

Munson, H. (2003, March). *Valuing experience: How to motivate and retain mature workers* (Report No. 1329-03-RR). New York: The Conference Board.

Nelson, T. D. (Ed.). (2002). *Ageism: Stereotyping and prejudice against older persons.* Cambridge, MA: MIT Press.

Newquist, D. D. (1986). Toward assessing health and functional capacity for policy development on work–life extension. In J. E. Birren, P. K. Robinson, & J. E. Livingston (Eds.), *Age, health, and employment* (pp. 27–44). Englewood Cliffs, NJ: Prentice-Hall.

Novelli, W. D. (2002, February). *How aging boomers will affect American business.* Paper presented at the meeting of The Wisemen, New York.

Older Americans Act of 1965, 42 U.S.C. § 3001 *et seq.* (2004).

Ones, D. S., & Viswesvaran, C. (1998). Gender, age and race differences on overt integrity tests: Analyses across four large-scale applicant data sets. *Journal of Applied Psychology, 83,* 35–42.

Organ, D. W. (1997). Organizational citizenship behavior: It's construct clean-up time. *Human Performance, 10,* 85–97.

Park, D. C. (1994). Aging, cognition, and work. *Human Performance, 7,* 181–205.

Parnes, H. S. (1988). The retirement decision. In M. E. Borus, H. S. Parnes, S. H. Sandell, & B. Seidman (Eds.), *The older worker* (pp. 115–150). Madison, WI: Industrial Relations Research Association.

Paul, C. E. (1988). Implementing alternative work arrangements for older work-ers. In H. Dennis (Ed.), *Fourteen steps in managing an aging work force* (pp. 113–119). Lexington, MA: Lexington Books.

Penner, R. G., Perun, P., & Steuerle, E. (2002). *Legal and institutional impediments to partial retirement and part-time work by older workers.* Washington, DC: Urban Institute.

The pension underfunding crisis: How effective have funding reforms been? Testimony before the Committee on Education and the Workforce, 108th Cong., 1 (2003) (testimony of D. C. John).

Perry, E. L., Kulik, C. T., & Bourhis, A. C. (1996). Moderating effects of personal and contextual factors in age discrimination. *Journal of Applied Psychology, 81,* 628–647.

Peterson, D. A., & Wendt, P. A. (1995). Training and education of older Ameri-cans as workers and volunteers. In S. A. Bass (Ed.), *Older and active: How Americans over 55 are contributing to society* (pp. 217–236). New Haven, CT: Yale University Press.

Peterson, P. G. (1999, January/February). Gray dawn: The global aging crisis. *Foreign Affairs, 78*(1), 42–55.

Preston, S. H., & Martin, L. G. (1994). Introduction. In L. G. Martin & S. H. Preston (Eds.), *Demography of aging* (pp. 1–7). Washington, DC: National Academy Press.

Quinn, J. F. (1999a, May). *Has the early retirement trend reversed?* Paper presented at the annual joint conference of the Retirement Research Consortia, Wash-ington, DC.

Quinn, J. F. (1999b, February). *Retirement patterns and bridge jobs in the 1990s* (EBRI Issue Brief No. 206). Washington, DC: Employee Benefit Research Institute.

Quinn, J. F., & Burkhauser, R. V. (1994). Retirement and labor force behavior of the elderly. In L. G. Martin & S. H. Preston (Eds.), *Demography of Aging* (pp. 56–61). Washington, DC: National Academy Press.

Rebick, M. (1993). The Japanese approach to finding jobs for older workers. In O. S. Mitchell (Ed.), *As the workforce ages: Costs, benefits, and policy chal-lenges* (pp. 103–124). Ithaca, NY: ILR Press.

Reynolds, C. A., Finkel, D., Gatz, M., & Pedersen, N. L. (2002). Sources of influ-ences on rate of cognitive change over time in Swedish twins: An applica-tion of latent growth models. *Experimental Aging Research, 28,* 407–433.

Rhodes, S. R. (1983). Age-related differences in work attitudes and behavior: A review and conceptual analysis. *Psychological Bulletin, 93,* 328–367.

Riemann, R., Angleitner, A., & Strelau, J. (1997). Genetic and environmental influences on personality: A study of twins reared together using the self- and peer report NEO–FFI scales. *Journal of Personality, 65*, 449–475.

Rix, S. E. (1990). *Older workers.* Santa Barbara, CA: ABC-CLIO.

Rix, S. E. (2001, November). *Toward active ageing in the 21st century: Working longer in the United States.* Paper prepared for the Japanese Institute of Labour Millennium Project, Tokyo, Japan. Retrieved February 8, 2003, from http://www.jil.go.jp/jil/seika/us2.pdf

Rix, S. (2002, April). *Update on the older worker.* Washington, DC: AARP Research Center.

Roberts, B. W., Caspi, A., & Moffitt, T. E. (2003). Work experiences and personality development in young adulthood. *Journal of Personality and Social Psychology, 84*, 582–593.

Roberts, B. W., Helson, R., & Klohnen, E. (2002). Personality development and growth in women across 30 years: Three perspectives. *Journal of Personality, 70*, 79–102.

Robson, W. B. P. (2001, October). *Aging populations and the workforce: Challenges for employers.* Winnipeg, Manitoba: British–North American Committee.

Rosen, B., & Jerdee, T. H. (1976). The nature of job-related age stereotypes. *Journal of Applied Psychology, 61*, 180–183.

Rosen, B., & Jerdee, T. H. (1977). Too old or not too old? *Harvard Business Review, 55*, 97–106.

Rosen, B., & Jerdee, T. H. (1985). *Older employees: New roles for valued resources.* Homewood, IL: Dow Jones-Irwin.

Rosow, J. M., & Zager, R. (1980). *The future of older workers in America: New perspectives for an extended work life.* Scarsdale, NY: Work in America Institute.

Ruhm, C. J. (1990). Career jobs, bridge employment, and retirement. In P. B. Doeringer (Ed.), *Bridges to retirement: Older workers in a changing labor market* (pp. 92–107). Ithaca, NY: ILR Press.

Ryff, C. D. (1989). Happiness is everything, or is it? Explorations on the meaning of psychological well-being. *Journal of Personality and Social Psychology, 57*, 1069–1081.

Ryff, C. D., & Keyes, C. L. M. (1995). The structure of psychological well-being revisited. *Journal of Personality and Social Psychology, 69*, 719–727.

Ryff, C. D., Kwan, C. M. L., & Singer, B. (2001). Personality and aging: Flourishing agendas and future challenges. In J. E. Birren & K. W. Schaie (Eds.), *Handbook of the psychology of aging* (5th ed., pp. 477–499). San Diego, CA: Academic Press.

Safire, W. (1977, October 3). The codgerdoggle. *New York Times*, p. 30.

Salthouse, T. A. (1984). Effects of age and skill in typing. *Journal of Experimental Psychology: General, 13*, 345–371.

Salthouse, T. A. (1990). Working memory as a processing resource in cognitive aging. *Developmental Review, 10*, 101–124.

Salthouse, T. A., Hambrick, D. Z., Lukas, K. E., & Dell, T. C. (1996). Determinants of adult age differences on synthetic work performance. *Journal of Experimental Psychology: Applied, 2*, 305–329.

Salthouse, T. A., & Maurer, J. J. (1996). Aging, job performance, and career development. In J. E. Birren & K. W. Schaie (Eds.), *Handbook of the psychology of aging* (4th ed., pp. 353–364). New York: Academic Press.

Schaie, K. W. (1983). The Seattle longitudinal study: A 21-year exploration of psychometric intelligence in adulthood. In K. W. Schaie (Ed.), *Longitudinal studies of adult psychological development* (pp. 31–44). New York: Springer Publishing Company.

Schaie K. W. (1984). Midlife influences upon intellectual functioning in old age. *International Journal of Behavioral Development, 7*, 463–478.

Schaie, K. W. (1989). Perceptual speed in adulthood: Cross-sectional and longitudinal studies. *Psychology and Aging, 4*, 443–453.

Schaie, K. W. (1993). The Seattle longitudinal studies of adult intelligence. *Current Directions in Psychological Science, 2*, 171–175.

Schaie, K. W. (1994). The course of adult intellectual development. *American Psychologist, 49*, 304–313.

Schaie, K. W., & Willis, S. L. (1986). Can intellectual decline in the elderly be reversed? *Developmental Psychology, 22*, 223–232.

Schappe, S. P. (1998). The influence of job satisfaction, organizational commitment, and fairness perceptions on organizational citizenship behavior. *Journal of Psychology, 132*, 277–290.

Schetagne, S. (2001). *Building bridges across generations in the workplace: A response to aging of the workforce* (Report No. 702). Vancouver, British Columbia, Canada: Columbia Foundation.

Schneider, B., Goldstein, H. W., & Smith, D. B. (1995). The ASA framework: An update. *Personnel Psychology, 40*, 747–773.

Schneider, B., Smith, D. B., Taylor, S., & Fleenor, J. (1998). Personality and organizations: A test of the homogeneity of personality hypothesis. *Journal of Applied Psychology, 83*, 462–470.

Schooler, C., Caplan, L., & Oates, G. (1998). Aging and work: An overview. In K. W. Schaie & C. Schooler (Eds.), *Impact of work on older adults* (pp. 1–19). New York: Springer Publishing Company.

Schooler, C., Mulatu, M. S., & Oates, G. (1999). The continuing effects of substantively complex work on the intellectual functioning of older workers. *Psychology and Aging, 14*, 483–506.

Scottish Council for Research in Education. (1933). *The intelligence of Scottish children: A national survey of an age-group.* London: University of London Press.

Shea, G. F. (1991). *Managing older employees.* San Francisco: Jossey-Bass.

Sheppard, H. L., & Rix, S. E (1977). *The graying of working America: The coming crisis in retirement-age policy.* New York: Free Press.

Shonk, J. H. (1992). *Team-based organizations: Developing a successful team environment.* Homewood IL: Business One Irwin.

Shultz, K. S. (2003). Bridge employment: Work after retirement. In G. A. Adams & T. A. Beehr (Eds.), *Retirement: Reasons, processes, and results* (pp. 214–241). New York: Springer Publishing Company.

Simon, R. (1996, July). Too damn old. *Money, 25*(7), 118–126.

Simpson, P. A., Greller, M. M., & Stroh, L. K. (2002). Variations in human capital investment activity by age. *Journal of Vocational Behavior, 61*, 109–138.

Singer, B. H., & Ryff, C. D. (1999). Hierarchies of life histories and associated health risks. In N. D. Adler, B. S. McEwen, & M. Marmot (Eds.), *Annals of the New York Academy of Sciences: Vol. 896. Socioeconomic status in industrialized countries* (pp. 96–115). New York: New York Academy of Sciences.

Siu, O.-L., Spector, P. E., Cooper, C. L., & Donald, I. (2001). Age differences in coping and locus of control: A study of managerial stress in Hong Kong. *Psychology and Aging, 16*, 707–710.

Smith v. City of Jackson, 351 U.S. 183 (2005).

Smith, P., Kendall, L., & Hulin, C. (1969). *The measurement of satisfaction of work and retirement.* Chicago: Rand McNally.

Social Security Act of 1935, 42 U.S.C. § 301 *et seq.* (2004).

Sonnenfeld, J. (1988). Continued work contributions in late career. In H. Dennis (Ed.), *Fourteen steps in managing an aging work force* (pp. 191–211). Lexington, MA: Lexington Books.

Sothmann, M. S., Saupe, K., Jasenof, D., & Blaney, J. (1992). Heart rate response of fire fighters to actual emergencies: Implications for cardiorespiratory fitness. *Journal of Occupational Medicine, 34*, 797–800.

Sparks, K., Faragher, B., & Cooper, C. L. (2001). Well-being and occupational health in the 21st century workplace. *Journal of Occupational and Organizational Psychology, 74*, 489–510.

Sparrow, P. R., & Davies, D. R. (1988). Effects of age, tenure, training, and job complexity on technical performance. *Psychology and Aging, 3*, 307–314.

Stagner, R. (1985). Aging in industry. In J. E. Birren & K. W. Schaie (Eds.), *Handbook of the psychology of aging* (pp. 798–817). New York: Van Nostrand Reinhold.

Steinhauser, S. (1998, July). Age bias: Is your corporate culture in need of an overhaul? *HR Magazine, 43*(8), 86–92.

Sterns, A. A., Sterns, H. L., & Hollis, L. A. (1996). The productivity and functional limitation of older adult workers. In W. Crown (Ed.), *Handbook on employment and the elderly* (pp. 276–303). Westport, CT: Greenwood Press.

Sterns, H. L. (1986). Training and retraining adult and older adult workers. In J. E. Birren, P. K. Robinson, & J. E. Livingston (Eds.), *Age, health, and employment* (pp. 93–113). Englewood Cliffs, NJ: Prentice-Hall.

Sterns, H. L. (1998). Commentary: The decision to retire or work. In K. W. Schaie & C. Schooler (Eds.), *Impact of work on older adults* (pp. 131–142). New York: Springer Publishing Company.

Sterns, H. L., & Alexander, R. A. (1987). Industrial gerontology: The aging individual and work. In K. Schaie (Ed.), *Annual review of gerontology and geriatrics* (pp. 93–113). New York: Springer Publishing Company.

Sterns, H. L., & Alexander, R. A. (1988). Performance appraisal of the older worker. In H. Dennis (Ed.), *Fourteen steps in managing an aging work force* (pp. 85–93). Lexington, MA: Lexington Books.

Sterns, H. L., Barrett, G. V., & Alexander, R. A. (1985). Accidents and the aging individual. In J. E. Birren & K. W. Schaie, *Handbook of the psychology of aging* (pp. 703–724). New York: Van Nostrand Reinhold.

Sterns, H. L., & Doverspike, D. (1988). Training and developing the older worker: Implications for human resource management. In H. Dennis (Ed.), *Fourteen steps in managing an aging work force* (pp. 97–110). Lexington, MA: Lexington Books.

Sterns, H. L., & Doverspike, D. (1989). Age and the training and learning process. In I. L. Goldstein (Ed.), *Training and development in organizations* (pp. 299–332). San Francisco: Jossey-Bass.

Sterns, H. L., Doverspike, D., & Lax, G. A. (2005). The Age Discrimination in Employment Act. In F. Landy (Ed.), *Employment discrimination litigation: Behavioral, quantitative, and legal perspectives* (pp. 256–293). San Francisco: Jossey-Bass.

Sterns, H. L., & Gray, J. D. (1999). Work, leisure, and retirement. In J. C. Cavanaugh & S. K. Whitbourne (Eds.), *Gerontology: An interdisciplinary perspective* (pp. 355–390). New York: Oxford University Press.

Sterns, H. L., & Huyck, M. H. (2001). The role of work in midlife. In M. E. Lachman (Ed.), *Handbook of midlife development* (pp. 447–486). New York: Wiley.

Sterns, H. L., & Kaplan, J. (2003). Self-management of career and retirement. In G. A. Adams & T. A. Beehr (Eds.), *Retirement: Reasons, processes, and results* (pp. 188–213). New York: Springer Publishing Company.

Sterns, H. L., & Miklos, S. M. (1995). The aging worker in a changing environment: Organizational and individual issues. *Journal of Vocational Behavior*, *47*, 248–268.

Sterns, H. L., & Patchett, M. (1984). Technology and the aging adult: Career development and training. In P. R. Robinson & J. E. Birren (Eds.), *Aging and technology* (pp. 261–277). New York: Plenum Press.

Sterns, H. L., & Sterns, A. A. (1995). Health and the employment capability of older Americans. In S. A. Bass (Ed.), *Older and active: How Americans over 55 are contributing to society* (pp. 10–34). New Haven, CT: Yale University Press.

Straka, G. A. (1998). Commentary: Organization, self-directed learning, and chronological age. In K. W. Schaie & C. Schooler (Eds.), *Impact of work on older adults* (pp. 186–194). New York: Springer Publishing Company.

Sum, A. M., & Fogg, W. N. (1990). Profile of the labor market for older workers. In P. B. Doeringer (Ed.), *Bridges to retirement: Older workers in a changing labor market* (pp. 33–63). Ithaca, NY: ILR Press.

Szinovacz, M. E. (2003). Contexts and pathways: Retirement as institution, process, and experience. In G. A. Adams & T. A. Beehr (Eds.), *Retirement: Reasons, processes, and results* (pp. 6–52). New York: Springer Publishing Company.

Tager, R. M. (1988). Stress and the older worker. In H. Dennis (Ed.), *Fourteen steps in managing an aging work force* (pp. 55–66). Lexington, MA: Lexington Books.

Taub, S. (2004, June 18). *Pension underfunding improves slightly.* Retrieved October 24, 2004, from www.cfo.com/article.cfm/3014679

Taylor, M. A., & Doverspike, D. (2003). Retirement planning and preparation. In G. A. Adams & T. A. Beehr (Eds.), *Retirement: Reasons, processes, and results* (pp. 53–82). New York: Springer Publishing Company.

Thomas, S. A., Browning, C. J., & Greenwood, K. M. (1994). Rehabilitation of older injured workers. *Disability and Rehabilitation, 16*, 162–170.

Thompson, L., Griffiths, A., & Davison, S. (2000). Employee absence, age and tenure: A study of nonlinear effects and trivariate models. *Work and Stress, 14*, 16–34.

Thornton, J. E. (2002). Myths of aging or ageist stereotypes. *Educational Gerontology, 28*, 301–312.

Toossi, M. (2002). A century of change: The U.S. labor force, 1950–2050. *Monthly Labor Review, 125*, 15–28.

Uccello, C. E. (1998, October). *Factors influencing retirement: Their implications for raising retirement age* (Public Policy Institute Report No. 9810). Washington, DC: AARP.

U.S. Department of Health and Human Services, Administration on Aging. (2001). *A profile of older Americans: 2001*. Washington, DC: Author.

U.S. Department of Health and Human Services, Administration on Aging. (2003). *Older population by age: 1900 to 2050*. Retrieved March 10, 2003, from http://www.aoa.gov/prof/statistics/online_stat_data/agepop2050.asp

U.S. Department of Labor, Bureau of Labor Statistics. (2001). *Economic and employment projections: 2000–2010*. Retrieved March 24, 2003, from http://www.bls.gov/emp

U.S. Department of Labor, Bureau of Labor Statistics. (2003). *Occupational outlook handbook*. Washington, DC: Author.

U.S. Department of Labor, Employee Benefits Security Administration. (2004, Summer). *Private Pension Plan Bulletin: Abstract of 1999 Form 5500 annual reports*. Available at www.dol.gov/ebsa/pdf/1999pensionplanbulletin.pdf

Vaillant, G. E. (2002). *Aging well*. Boston: Little, Brown & Company.

Waldman, D. A., & Avolio, B. J. (1986). A meta-analysis of age differences in job performance. *Journal of Applied Psychology, 71*, 33–38.

Walker, A. (1999). Combating age discrimination in the workplace. *Experimental Aging Research, 25*, 367–378.

Warr, P. (1994). Age and employment. In H. C. Triandis, M. D. Dunnette, & L. M. Hough (Eds.), *Handbook of industrial and organizational psychology* (2nd ed., Vol. 4, pp. 485–550). Palo Alto, CA: Consulting Psychologists Press.

Warr, P. (1998). Age, work, and mental health. In K. W. Schaie & C. Schooler (Eds.), *Impact of work on older adults* (pp. 252–303). New York: Springer Publishing Company.

Warr, P. (2001). Age and work behaviour: Physical attributes, cognitive abilities, knowledge, personality traits, and motives. *International Review of Industrial and Organizational Psychology, 16*, 1–36.

Warr, P., Miles, A., & Platts, C. (2001). Age and personality in the British population between 16 and 64 years. *Journal of Occupational and Organizational Psychology, 74*, 165–199.

Weckerle, J. R., & Schultz, K. S. (1999). Influences on the bridge employment decision among older USA workers. *Journal of Occupational and Organizational Psychology, 72*, 317–329.

Wellner, A. S. (2002, March). Tapping a silver mine. *HR Magazine, 47*(3), pp. 26–32.

Whalley, L. J., & Deary, I. J. (2001). Longitudinal cohort study of childhood IQ and survival up to age 76. *British Medical Journal, 322*, 1–5.

Wiatrowski, W. J. (2001). Changing retirement age: Ups and downs. *Monthly Labor Review, 124*, 3–12.

Wiatrowski, W. J. (2004). Medical and retirement plan coverage: Exploring the decline in recent years. *Monthly Labor Review, 127*, 29–36.

Williams, S., & Shaw, W. T. (1999). Mood and organizational citizenship behavior: The effects of positive affect on employee organizational citizenship behavior intentions. *Journal of Psychology, 133*, 656–668.

Williamson, J. B., & McNamara, T. K. (2001, November). *Why some workers remain in the labor force beyond the typical age of retirement* (CRR WP 2001-09). Chestnut Hill, MA: Center for Retirement Research at Boston College.

Willis, S. L., & Schaie, K. W. (1986). Training the elderly on the ability factors of spatial orientation and inductive reasoning. *Psychology and Aging, 1*, 239–247.

Wineman, J. (1988). Age issues in the workplace: A labor perspective. In H. Dennis (Ed.), *Fourteen steps in managing an aging work force* (pp. 173–187). Lexington, MA: Lexington Books.

Workforce Investment Act of 1998, 29 U.S.C. § 936 *et seq.* (2000).

Yeatts, D. L., Folts, W. E., & Knapp, J. (2000). Older workers' adaptation to a changing workplace: Employment issues for the 21st century. *Educational Gerontology, 26*, 566–582.

Zimfrich, P. (2002). Cross-sectionally and longitudinally balanced effects of processing speed on intellectual abilities. *Experimental Aging Research, 28*, 231–251.

Zink, D. L. (2002, July). Improvidently granted: The Supreme Court hesitates. *The Industrial–Organizational Psychologist, 40*, 96–98.

Index

About the Authors

Jerry W. Hedge, PhD, has been involved in personnel research for more than 25 years. He has worked with a wide variety of clients designing, implementing, and evaluating numerous organizational tools, systems, and techniques. During his career, Dr. Hedge has stayed actively involved in publishing his research and presenting regularly at professional conferences. He is a fellow of the Society for Industrial and Organizational Psychology and the American Psychological Association. He received his PhD in industrial–organizational psychology from Old Dominion University, Norfolk, Virginia.

Walter C. Borman, PhD, is currently the chief executive officer of Personnel Decisions Research Institutes, Tampa, Florida, and professor of industrial–organizational psychology at the University of South Florida. He is a fellow of the Society for Industrial and Organizational Psychology (SIOP), and in 1994–1995 served as president of the society. Dr. Borman has written more than 300 books, book chapters, journal articles, and conference papers, and he was the recipient of SIOP's Distinguished Scientific Contributions Award for 2003. He received his PhD in industrial–organizational psychology from the University of California, Berkeley.

Steven E. Lammlein, PhD, is an industrial–organizational psychologist with 27 years of experience in human resources research and consulting. He has consulted with a large variety of private- and public-sector clients, and his work has addressed workforce issues in a wide variety of jobs across the occupational spectrum. His specialty areas include personnel selection and placement, certification testing, equal employment opportunity issues, job and training needs analysis, management development and succession planning, training design and evaluation, and performance management. He received his PhD from the University of Minnesota, Twin Cities.